The Madness of Our Lives

Experiences of mental breakdown and recovery

Penny Gray

Foreword by Peter Campbell

Jessica Kingsley Publishers
London and Philadelphia

Extract on p.6 from
Harpe

permission of

www.jkp.com

Library of Congress Cataloging in Publication Data
A CIP catalog record for this book is available from the Library of Congress

British Library Cataloguing in Publication Data
A CIP catalogue record for this book is available from the British Library

ISBN-13: 978 1 84310 057 7
ISBN-10: 1 84310 057 6

Printed and bound in Great Britain by
Athenaeum Press, Gateshead, Tyne and Wear

In memory of Lesley

Nervous breakdowns can be highly underrated
methods of spiritual transformation.
They certainly get your attention.

Marianne Williamson, A Return to Love

Contents

FOREWORD   9

ACKNOWLEDGEMENTS   10

INTRODUCTION   11

Part One: Dealing with life stresses

1. Eating a Mars bar: Jane Pole-Jones   17

2. Counselling was the turning point: Cheryl Stromeyer   34

3. No easy answers: Keith Bright   47

4. My music saved my life: Julie O'Connor   60

Part Two: Women survivors of childhood abuse

5. I was lucky in a way: Steph Corby   79

6. I'd always thought crying was a sin: Diane Johnson   96

7. Oops, there goes the telly: Lesley Tutt   108

Part Three: Young men in crisis

8.   I'd rather it was a chapter I'd forgotten about: Paul Mann   127

9.   Doing all right, considering: Adrian Stiles   138

10. It does teach you a bit about human nature: Graeme Wilson   146

Part Four: An insider perspective

11. Really enthusiastic about antidepressants:
     Stephen Goodfellow   157

     Postscript   175

     The professional view   176

     Conclusions and practical advice   189

     REFERENCES   200

     FURTHER READING   201

     RESOURCES   202

Foreword

Madness remains a taboo in most contemporary societies. Although we may think we have placed it under more effective control – by talking of mental illness not madness, by appointing an array of mental health professionals with supposed expertise in the supervision and treatment of people with a mental illness diagnosis – we do not wish to be too closely associated with mad people or to know too much about the realities of their lives.

But we need to change – for our own sakes and for the sakes of people who suffer the deep-rooted discrimination attached to a mental illness diagnosis. For these modern citizens no longer live behind the walls of remote and closely regulated asylums, but alongside us in the communities where we work and play. They are fighting for the same rights we enjoy.

Building better community mental health services will not be sufficient. Service users are social agents now. Only changes in social attitudes and practices will secure them the position they deserve. Real change must involve education to lead ourselves out of the suspicion, prejudice and fear we have inherited. In particular, we need to listen to the voices and stories of those with direct experience of mental illness/madness. They can show us the true dimensions of their lives. They can reveal that it is possible to live through the turmoil of mental distress.

In recent years, the voices of such people have won greater respect. As one of them and one of us, I warmly welcome this anthology of personal testimony.

Peter Campbell, Founder member of Survivors Speak Out and Survivors' Poetry

Acknowledgements

I am deeply indebted to my contributors for sharing their stories. I have many times found myself moved to tears or anger working on the texts. This book is a tribute to the courage and generosity of these folks – I have tried my best to do it justice.

Grateful thanks to Tony Parker, whose book, *The Violence of Our Lives: Interviews with Life-Sentence Prisoners in America*, inspired the title of this one, as well as the story chapter format.

Sincere thanks also to Andy Ward and Peter Campbell for consistent good support, advice and encouragement. Jan Wallcraft, Phil Thomas, Alison Faulkner, Piers Allott, Mick Carpenter, Jim Read, George Monbiot, Anna Thornhill, Chris Vezey, Fran Shall and Maggie Black were also generous with their time and energy. Thank you too to many friends and family members for their kindness, consideration and forbearance during the years it has taken to get this into print – and special thanks to Paul Kirkley.

Finally, I am grateful to BBC Radio 4 for permission to use parts of an interview broadcast in their series 'Tuesday Lives', and to Manchester Mind for their permission to use an extract from an article written by one of my contributors for their magazine, *Mindfield*.

Penny Gray

Introduction

Mental distress affects everyone. Far less commonly does it progress to mental breakdown, and since mental breakdown is a lay term rather than a medical one, there are no statistics on prevalence. Yet it is probably fair to say that almost everyone knows someone who has been affected. And because mental breakdown is stigmatising and not generally talked about, it is also a fair bet that there is more of it around than most of us are aware of. This book is an attempt to put that right.

The story of the book starts with my own. I suffered a mental breakdown in my early twenties, shortly after finishing my undergraduate degree at university. For years I had been extremely anxious about exams, and my finals were no exception. I had a place lined up at medical school, and I was feeling sick all the way through. I thought there was a possibility that I might be pregnant, but I didn't want to look at it: I had to focus on my revision.

After my finals were over I went to the student health centre and had a pregnancy test, which was positive. I was stunned and confused by the news. I didn't want to tell my parents, and besides, I had set my heart on med school and a baby would have been the end of it. So I ended up in hospital. One in three women has a termination of pregnancy at some stage, apparently. Why don't we hear more about it? Certainly, nothing prepared me for the trauma of it all.

I was four, five weeks into my first term at medical school when I started to lose it. I stopped eating, stopped sleeping, and all the hurt and anger I had been suppressing came bubbling up to the surface. I was angry that I hadn't been properly warned about the high risk of pregnancy with an IUD at that age, angry that the termination had been presented as a minor medical procedure, easily justified on health grounds, and angry that I'd never been offered any counselling or support. And I was full of remorse. I gradually stopped going in for lectures at college. I was very distraught, and I was upsetting others.

The actual breakdown – the acute phase of my grieving process – lasted for five or six weeks. I ended up in the middle of the night one night, feeling totally abandoned, having hit rock bottom. I had borrowed my mother's car a few days before, and I got into the car and drove it to Oxford – for no particular reason other than I saw a road sign and I had always fancied going there. I slept in the car for a couple of hours when I arrived, and then I walked around for the rest of the day in a daze, going nowhere in particular. I ended up sitting on a bench on that sunny autumn afternoon, having exhausted all my resources, feeling totally empty. I was looking at the wind blowing through some trees, and somehow I noticed how beautiful it all was. In that moment, something shifted: it was as if I had fallen right through all the grief and the pain, and into a space of emptiness and peace. It was a remarkably powerful, beautiful contrast to the trauma of the previous weeks, and its impact has stayed with me since.

I don't know how long I was sitting on that bench, but I got up a different person. Not that my difficulties were over – they weren't. It took nearly a year to put my life back together. Pretty quickly, I went to see my tutor and resigned from medical school. For months I was very down-hearted about the termination, which was the hardest part. But I always felt lucky to have escaped involvement with the mental health services, and lucky too to have had good support from family and friends, and resources enough to take a year out from my postgraduate studies.

The experience cemented a life-long fascination with mind and mental health, and I determined in the long term to look at these issues more deeply, and to talk to others about their experiences of breakdown and recovery. It took me many years to get to a place where I was ready to do this, and longer still to find the time. Finally I was able to start when I went freelance in 1993. I began by volunteering at a local Mind drop-in centre. Soon afterwards I started to teach re-evaluation counselling – a form of peer counselling in which people learn to listen to and counsel each other to function more effectively in their lives. In parallel, I advertised for people to come forward with their own stories of mental breakdown and recovery.

I collected the stories that make up this book over a 13-month period in 1994–95. Altogether I interviewed 14 people, the only criteria being that they should have had a mental breakdown and should consider themselves recovered. Six of my contributors were recruited directly through an advertisement in the bi-monthly newsletter of Survivors Speak Out, a

London-based organisation consisting mostly of mental health service user activists interested in improving the mental health system and people's attitudes towards service users. Two contributors were friends of one of these 'Survivors'; four others were personal contacts; and two were doctors I recruited through a personal advertisement in the *British Medical Journal*. Most of the interviews took place at the contributors' homes, and lasted two to three hours.

Out of the 14 stories I selected 11 that I thought would give the most representative and readable mix for a compilation. Effectively this meant that I de-selected three – all for essentially the same reason – that they overlapped with those that I decided to include, such that leaving them out would not detract from the general drift, and I needed to restrict inclusion for reasons of space.

Listening to my contributors' stories at the time was deeply fascinating and not too shocking for me. I had by then done a lot of co-counselling and heard a lot of horror stories. Besides which, I warmed to each person as I listened to them. This was at least partly because I identified with so much of their experience each time. Working with the stories was far more difficult than I expected. Technically, it involved editing them to a half or a third of their original length, cutting out the repetition within and between stories, and trimming details that were not strictly necessary to the flow and the sense. This was time-consuming but not hard. But beyond this, I frequently found the material very moving and at times disturbing – much more so than I had done at interview, surprisingly.

In editing the transcripts, I have tried to remain strictly true to the words and spirit of each person's story. Nothing has been added by me, with the exception of the odd linking word to give continuity to a thread. At the start of each story I have included a thumbnail of my initial contact with the person, giving a few background details about them; their age, what they do for a living, how they first came into contact with the mental health services and so on – to provide some context. Where possible I sent the stories back to the speakers for review, making minor changes on request at this point regarding issues of confidentiality. Names and other key details have been changed for the same reason.

Being such a limited number, these accounts cannot hope to give a complete picture of the experiences of breakdown and strategies for recovery in the wider population; nor is this their aim. The intention is rather to present a series of snapshots or short films, giving just a few insider perspectives on mental distress and the mental health services in parallel. From these I hope to highlight the common threads, with a view to seeing what contributes both to keeping someone stuck in their distress and to helping them to recover from it.

My contributors come from a range of different backgrounds and life experiences, as their stories testify. I have ordered the chapters in a way that emphasises the similarities between some of the different stories on the basis of what caused each person's breakdown. This of course is a personal view, but I hope it will be helpful.

Following the stories, I have included a chapter presenting the views of a few, more user-centred mental health workers. This chapter, again, is based on one-to-one interviews, only this time with five individuals who have worked for many years in mental health, and who might be considered fairly radical in their perspectives compared with the mainstream. I wanted to include these to give an alternative take on recovery and on the mental health services – views that might differ from those of many who work within the services, as well as myself and my contributors. Jan Wallcraft and Alison Faulkner are ser-vice-user consultants: Jan was working for the Sainsbury Centre for Mental Health and Alison was at the Mental Health Foundation when we met. Dr Phil Thomas is a former consultant psychiatrist who preferred to work outside the medical model; he has also been a regular contributor to *Open Mind* magazine, the bi-monthly magazine of the mental health charity, Mind. Mick Carpenter is a reader/researcher in social policy at the University of Warwick, and Piers Allott was at the time Strategic Policy Advisor to the Department of Health on recovery from mental health problems.

The final chapter discusses the common threads and themes that unite the stories, focusing in particular on the central importance of self-management in recovery and the implications for mental health practice.

The terms 'breakdown' and 'recovery' are defined by the speakers throughout.

PART ONE
Dealing with life stresses

1.

Eating a Mars bar: Jane Pole-Jones

I went to meet Jane at her family home: a picturesque thatched cottage in an orchard garden. It's the genuine article: low-beamed ceilings, polished wood floors and oriental carpets. Jane too has an attractive character; she's in her forties, slim, articulate, and bright-eyed. Passing her in the street, it would never cross your mind that she spent nearly 22 years in and out of psychiatric hospitals, first with anorexia and then with an apparent psychotic illness. She seems perfectly fine now: married with a son who's living at home, she draws, paints and reads in her spare time. Her problems began when she was a teenager in the sixties.

Here's a cutting from the *Evening Post*, which is a local paper, and this was taken when I was at school. It's a picture of me posed very tweely among some trees and the caption is 'Nothing plain about this Jane'. It says, 'Here's one Jane who is far from being plain, she is Jane Ellis', that's my maiden name, '17, she's seen here in a rare moment of leisure, for when she is not at school studying English and classics, she is taking part in drama and music or indulging in a spot of fencing. Her ambition, to go to university to study law.' This amazing picture of this provocative looking girl.

Just beside it, as a matter of contrast, is a picture taken a couple of years later and this is an appalling face, like a skull really; the eyes are staring out, almost like mad eyes, and my neck is scrawny and old like a 90-year old's. As you can see, it's one of those stomach-churning photos that makes you feel a bit ill when you look at it. I weighed about five stone then. I can remember very very clearly always being aware of the fact that I had to be good; very very good, not just a little bit good, but perfectly good. I was very academically conscientious, the only girl at my little village school who passed the 11-plus and went up to the grammar school, I worked really hard, very anxious to please. I had lots of boyfriends, I mean not just a few, but I was overwhelmed with them really. I was good at sport, I could swim, I was head girl, I was chairman of the Debating Society, there wasn't a thing that I didn't shine at and yet, if you'd have said to me, are you good at any of these things, I'd have said no I'm not, not good enough, not good enough. I think that's always what I thought about myself, that I shall never ever be good enough at anything. My life was getting a bit out of control with all this trying to please people.

★ ★ ★

I think I was coping until 1967 when Twiggy came in, and everybody in the class, every single person, decided to go on a diet. Of course in those days we didn't know about calories, so we just boycotted school lunches. And literally within the first two days of stopping eating, I started to feel absolutely wonderful. I'd say I became anorectic almost on the first day. It was almost as if I'd taken total control of myself. I felt completely elated, powerful and strong and it became an absolute addiction to maintain this regime, it became my raison d'être, my identity. After about six months all the worries and problems of my life evaporated, because all I thought about was how I was going to avoid eating the next meal. But unfortunately as it went on it also polarised my intellectual activity, I found it harder and harder to study, and as the weight began to drop off other people began to notice and it soon became obvious, well I suppose about 18 months later, that this magnificent cop-out I'd found was going to be taken away from me. Of course by this time I was looking very ill and my work was suffering.

In the end my parents took me to see an endocrinologist. I think he knew what was wrong as soon as he saw me. He started off by doing barium meals and things, and eventually he said, 'I think your daughter's got this problem called anorexia'. Nobody had heard of it. He gave me Largactil and insulin coma, now this was a endocrinologist, not a psychiatrist. And he gave me Valium. This was in the general hospital, just in the two weeks I was in there to be assessed. And I kept going into comas every morning because the nurses didn't know they were supposed to give me breakfast, they were giving me insulin, a perfectly healthy person. But the worst thing was the Largactil because it just transformed me; I became an instant vegetable. I couldn't read, couldn't do anything – I felt absolutely awful. I didn't associate it with the medicine, because they hadn't told me what it was, they just said, 'Take this tablet, you'll feel better'.

After a while I came out. I carried on taking the drugs but I had to literally force myself around. In the end my GP, who was getting a bit cross with all this, called in a psychiatrist for a second opinion, and this bloke from the local psychiatric hospital came to see me and he said to my parents, 'Yes, your daughter has anorexia, but she shouldn't be taking these drugs, she should come into the therapeutic community I've just opened and she'll be all right. She's just verging on it really and she'll be fine if we do this'. Of course my parents refused. They just didn't want to hear the words 'loony bin'. They absolutely wouldn't have anything to do with it. Instead they touted around London to all the various teaching hospitals to see if they could get me in to see somebody, and they ended up at St Thomas' with a very eminent professor of psychiatry. He was absolutely notorious in his day. He'd pioneered the idea that mental illness was physical. That all lunatic asylums, etc., should be banned, and that the only way to treat mental illness was with a very, very heavy drug regime.

He offered me an appointment and my parents took me up there. I can remember it to this day because he was the most hideous looking man, he looked like a frog, and he had a terrifying physical presence, very tall, big, powerful, awesome, very very frightening. He dragged me into this room and I looked up and there was a whole group of medical students. I sat there behind him as he spoke about me in the third person, this girl this and this girl that and she does this and she does that. I don't remember taking a lot of it in, but he fired questions at me, and then he told me to take all my clothes off. They were all male students, obviously, because it was 1967, and he stood with a stick and he pointed out the effects of starvation, just as if I was a piece of meat. It was terribly humiliating and quite wrong, and I lost my good manners, I think I said something. And he said, 'We're not going to be able to cope with somebody who flings their weight about like this, are we?' And they all laughed; they laughed at me. It was horrible, frightening, really.

★ ★ ★

I went up to his unit for psychiatric treatment. All the new drugs, the neuroleptics, had just starting coming in from the States, and everybody was very excited about them. The first thing he said to me was, 'These drugs are very important to you, you will probably have to take them for the rest of your life. You *must not ever* stop taking these drugs'. My parents drank all this in because he didn't mention being mad and it was all very respectable, nurses in white uniforms and so on.

Talk about feeding! I've had fattening up regimes since then, but this was 8000 calories a day, it was just food en masse. I had insulin coma every morning. I had ECT every other day. And I was on *4000 mg* of Largactil a day. Four thousand! The normal dose now is 400 mg for big men *in extremis*. I was on monoamine oxidase inhibitors, antidepressants, I was on tricyclic antidepressants. And then I had Melleril, and I had an injection as well, and obviously also Disipal to stop all the shaking. This was what we were given and put into bed, just lobotomised by drugs. You just slept, you could just about carry on a conversation while all this food was being pumped in. I kept slipping into comas every morning with this insulin treatment, but they never stopped it. I was always in intensive care. It was just an onslaught of chemicals.

When I came out I was a completely strange shape. I was barrelled with tiny skinny legs because I hadn't got out of bed for two months. I felt awful. I could hardly speak. I was so drugged up that I couldn't function on any level other than survival. And it hadn't taught me anything about food, I'd not resolved anything. And so it carried on. I had to take the tablets and go up as an outpatient. I had to carry on having ECT. I think over the next year I had a hundred ECTs in that room. My mother used to say, 'You were so much better when you had the ECT'. Because I just used to sit. To their mind I was restored to normal weight, so I was OK.

★　★　★

Then I went to Bristol University because my parents had managed to wangle me a place there doing English and drama. I don't know how I got through the first term really. It was ridiculous. On all this medication I couldn't go to lectures, couldn't read, because I couldn't focus – my eyes had gone funny with the Largactil. I couldn't keep awake, couldn't do anything really. I couldn't go out in the sunlight because the Largactil affects the skin. Didn't eat. So after the end of the first term I went back into St Thomas' again to be fattened up, and had more of the same.

After I came out the second time I started to do temp jobs and I just began to disintegrate. The jobs were all cleaning tables, washing up, I couldn't really manage anything else. I went in and out of hospital several times, seeing the same doctor. Around that time he said to my parents that he didn't think I had anorexia at all; I was a manic depressive. That meant that the drugs had to be slightly different, but the same thing really. And then he told them I was schizophrenic and they began to lose faith, because they didn't want to hear that, you know, that I was really mad.

Eventually my parents found me another doctor, a psychotherapist who was quite good actually, very supportive, but he had a problem with me in that by the time he saw me I'd become very strange. I think he was frightened to take me off the medication, so he cut it down quite a lot, and he said he thought I should move away from home. He was the head of a big mentally handicapped hospital and he said he could get me a job there as a nursing assistant and I'd live in the nurses' home. I think he wanted to see if just moving away from home would enable me to start functioning again, but I actually gave up eating altogether and then drinking, and my weight went down to its lowest yet, four and a half stone. I suppose within about four months I was obviously going to die. I couldn't walk up steps, it would take me 20 minutes to get up a flight of three steps and I was staggering along. By this time I wasn't eating anything at all. I had got to that stage of anorexia where you really can just die of starvation. So he admitted me to the local psychiatric hospital in Oxford, and that was where everything really started to go wrong for me.

★ ★ ★

First of all they started upping the Largactil. And then they wanted to give me ECT. Well I'd actually had enough of ECT, and this was the first bit of defiance I'd really ever shown. I said, 'I'm not having ECT'. They said, 'You've got to have ECT'. And I said, 'Well, I'm going to discharge myself then', and I went home. They'd give me large quantities of drugs and of course I hadn't got them at home so I started to withdraw from them. And I can remember running down the road, searching. I had this overwhelming feeling that there was going to be a wonderful party for me because I'd arrived, then the next thing I knew my mother had called the doctor and the social worker in and I was being shipped back to hospital under a compulsory section. Which was the first time I'd been sectioned. First of many.

By the time I got on the ambulance going back I'd started to hallucinate really badly, and it was actually very disgusting. Just before I discharged myself I'd started to eat in a rather frenzied manner because I think I'd realised that I was going to die, and my bowels weren't functioning so I began to get terrible diarrhoea which I couldn't control, and I began to freak out. So when we got to the hospital they gave me a massive injection of something or other and put me in the padded cell, no clothes, obviously. I'd got this terrible diarrhoea and it was just running everywhere and I didn't know what to do, there was nothing in there to clean it up, and I can remember them shouting at me that I was an animal, and filthy, that sort of thing. Which was true – I mean I couldn't deny it. I was I suppose a very obscene looking human being at this stage. I was a skeleton whose body was out of control and I was ranting, my hair had all fallen out and my gums were all swollen and bleeding, I was absolutely gross I suppose the word would be. And when I was there I had a massive fit. I remember suddenly feeling as if a huge explosion was happening in my brain and I saw the Virgin Mary and the angels and like a nativity scene, choirs and exaltation, it was; I saw it, I heard it, it was there in the room and I was being blessed, and I felt as if some sort of wonderful transformation had occurred within my brain. I'd flipped my lid basically.

I think I was in that cell for about three weeks. After they realised I'd had this fit they didn't give me ECT, but they put me back on the drugs as soon as they could and they kept me locked up without my clothes. It was when behaviour modification was coming in, and they started to do behaviour therapy with me. The drugs made me very dry, and I used to ask for water and they used to pour it down the sink in front of me to make me plead and beg for the water. They used to do the same thing with food. They used to throw it at me and make me grovel on the floor for it. They tried to force you into a position where you have to acknowledge that you are wrong. At one time they got two or three members of staff to rub mashed potato in my hair – it's absolutely unbelievable when you think about it now, and it was cruel. The whole thing was like a nightmare.

★ ★ ★

Anyway I'd got the idea that a device had been put inside my head and that I was going to be used for great scientific experiments connected with this device, and I began to see all this as a sort of benevolence. And I became totally weird, seriously weird. I'd made the connection that the drugs were controlling the device in my head which was relaying information back to the doctors who were putting it all into a big computer bank. I felt as if all my movements were being controlled and I was going to be a very important person, you know, tell them all they needed to know about the brain and the way it functioned. I felt very much as if the whole world had been set up for me, as if I was walking through a series of plays that had rehearsed and I was just playing my part. I used to get messages from the television; I would switch on the radio and it would be talking to me; and I would walk into a library and pick up a book and inside the book there would be a message for me, telling me what I had been thinking a minute previously. It was totally credible and I believed it, I believed that I had been singled out, and it gave me a sense of identity that I hadn't ever had. And even when I was four and a half stone I considered that I was totally and utterly sane – I was the only person in this madhouse who knew what they were doing – although I never spoke about my fantasy because that would have been to have spoilt my cover.

After quite a long time the psychotherapist managed to get me out, but I was under a lot of drugs again and I took a couple of overdoses, really quite dramatic ones with this heavy medication, not because I wanted to kill myself but because these internal voices told me that that was what I should do, you know, hang on, let's experiment in stomach wash-out and give you a try at this. But eventually I got my weight back to normal, and this doctor was good in that he encouraged me, he said, 'You know, you can look all right, you can do other things, you should join a club and see if you can meet a man'. By then I thought that he was controlling the experiment. He'd become a sort of Prospero to me, he was manipulating me, and I thought that he was doing it with hypnosis. But he was nice to me, very understanding. He even said nice things occasionally. Absolutely incredible. And he did enable me to put on weight, because I used the feeling that I was being controlled to get myself – bits of myself – sorted out. So I got my weight back to normal, and I looked less mad. I went and joined an intervarsity club, and there I met Tom, my husband; he was on the door at this meeting. I met him and a week later he proposed. Of course I thought this was all part of the experiment because he's a scientist, he's a physicist you see, and a man of very few words; he's not the sort of bloke that says 'I love you, I think you are wonderful'. So I thought he was just part of the experiment, and I married him thinking that he'd married me solely to control and manipulate the complicated controls in my brain. It didn't occur to me that he didn't know what was going on.

Poor old Tom, we'd only been married three days and I took an overdose. I mean, he knew that I was slightly unstable, but I think he was a bit besotted with me really, because I was looking quite nice by then and what have you. He had no idea.

★ ★ ★

Things were quite good really for a couple of years. I saw the doctor on and off most of the time, and he managed to keep me stable. I took Stelazine and Tryptizol and my Mogadon at night, that type of thing. I was still mad, still convinced that the whole world was an experiment, but I could actually manage to function enough to do a basic job. I don't suppose anybody meeting me would have thought I was anything particularly different, you know, but I used to find life very hard, it was like living on two dimensions; inside there would be all this madness, and then there was what I call coping, I've always coped, and this is really what throws people because they see this person who is obviously coping and yet is exceedingly mad. Then Tom got a job up in Scotland and we moved up there and I lost contact with my doctor. It was fine to start with. And then I wanted a baby. Or I should say, the computer in my head said, 'You've got to have a baby'.

★ ★ ★

I didn't really get on very well with the pregnancy. I developed high blood pressure within the first couple of months and I became more and more stressed out and they put me into hospital, I suppose when I was about five months pregnant, and I had to spend the whole time lying in bed in a darkened room, as you do with high blood pressure. I got quite panicky towards the end. They tried to induce this baby and it wouldn't come because all the drugs I was on had stopped the hormones functioning. So I had a Caesarian section, and they gave me massive amounts of pethidine. Well, pethidine makes anybody mad, and as I came around from having the anaesthetic I had a very big flare-up of what I now see was psychotic illness, and I started to rant and rave and accuse people of planting the baby on me; I was really mad, verbally mad. I was not only hallucinating like I normally did, but I was letting everybody know I was hallucinating, which was a little frightening, because it was a tiny Scottish hospital. After six weeks I went into a loony bin up in Scotland with Matthew, my baby, who was absolutely fine – 9 lbs, no problem.

★ ★ ★

I coped very well with Matthew really. He was in the bin with me for the first four months, and it was quite nice. They had a little mother and baby unit. Being an anorectic I did everything properly, and Matthew was given the best care. But there was absolutely no bond between us, he was just something that I did things to. I couldn't feel anything, I mean I had no emotions whatsoever. I think that is the most overbearing thing – since I was 16 I hadn't felt an emotion. I was just zombified. Then I was discharged and I became a revolving door [patient]. The drugs made me feel bad, I'd go back in, get discharged, the drugs made me feel bad, I'd go back in.

After the third time they wouldn't have Matthew in, so I had to go without him, which was very distressing, and I stopped eating. That was very easy because the food was really disgusting in that Scottish lunatic asylum. It was the worst food I have ever not eaten in my life. And as soon as I stopped eating I began to feel much better in myself, and of course I started to lose weight and went into another anorectic episode. I lost weight extremely quickly, and it wasn't very long before I was down to six stone and then everyone started to panic. Tom didn't know what to do really, I had this little boy and I was so drugged up and the weight was just falling off me, so he got a transfer back down to England again.

★　★　★

I got a place to see a renowned professor who had a clinic specifically designed for treating anorexia nervosa. Tom went in first for an hour, and I sat there getting more and more uptight. Then I went in for an hour. There was this man sitting there like a god, very erudite. I was at that level of functioning with drugs and starvation that I just couldn't understand what he was talking about, really – he spoke in, to my mind, riddles. He said, 'You know you have anorexia nervosa very severely', which I knew. And he said, 'I'm not sure about the other thing.' He said, 'It's very complicated'. I think by the other thing he meant schizophrenia. He said, 'I'm going to admit you into my unit, but we won't talk about the other thing, it'll be our secret'. So I immediately thought, 'Oh, he's part of the experiment, I'm not allowed to tell anybody the experiment is going on' – I just took it as collusion. But he also said that he wasn't going to take me off the drugs. Now this is a man who prided himself on running a drug-free unit. He said that he didn't think that I had schizophrenia, but he wasn't going to take me off the drugs, he wasn't prepared to take that level of risk.

Now if you really want to know about human abuses you want to spend three months in a ward like that being treated for anorexia. It's the whole bit: it's the little cubicle; it's not coming out for three months, it's one bath a week, supervised; performing on a commode and having it inspected. It's being in prison, having every human right taken away from you and being told that it's therapeutic and that it's got to raise your self-esteem. I think all psychiatric medicine is punitive. But this is punishment par excellence. I mean you wouldn't treat mass murderers like they treated those women.

I spent six months in that place. There were six anorectics in little cubicles. You didn't walk anywhere, you were wheeled on a wheelchair. You had one bath a week and one hair wash a week, you were allowed one bowl of water in the evening to wash yourself with and that was it. You weren't allowed any visitors unless your weight went up to a certain level. You were supposed to spend most of your time lying down, and if you didn't gain weight at a certain rate your privileges were taken away. Now I'd got a two-year-old little boy who was being looked after jointly by my mother and my husband, and I wasn't allowed to see him, he was used as a sort of bargaining chip. So I was very compliant. I knew what eating was all about: you go into a bin and you eat, you go out and you lose weight and you go in again. That was my philosophy, so I didn't worry about the food.

What annoyed me about the place is that you were told that you were going to get all this therapy and therapy amounted to a doctor who was on a three-month residency – I mean they were training doctors, they were there for three months, then they went on elsewhere. They used to come, they used to look at their watch, and they used to say, 'Oh, I've got 40 minutes'. Quite often they didn't turn up, or they weren't interested and they looked completely bored. The whole idea with therapists is that you should see them consistently over a length of time, and these were people who were frankly not interested, they were doing it because they'd been told to do it, and they put me down as being a vegetable anyway because I was on drugs. As far as I could see the therapeutic content was nil. And of course when you are in the bin most of the time is spent trying to get to see the doctor, because you go in and then you don't see a doctor for weeks and weeks and weeks, and sometimes you actually wonder if you are ever going to see one again.

We had these dreadful group therapy sessions, which was stupid really. You get a whole load of anorectics together all trying to be the thinnest, which is what it's about – I mean anorexics anyway have to be the best in every single aspect of their life – not in a competitive sense with other people, but with themselves. It was quite bizarre. And we had other people who were sick in there, it was a called a therapeutic community, and it was very intense. Everybody used to act out the whole time, everybody was forever slitting their wrists and stuffing pills down them, very inward looking. We weren't taught to relate to the outside world at all.

★ ★ ★

I didn't see many people getting well, I saw a lot of people getting very overwrought and picking up ideas from other people. Girls that had gone in there like myself, with pure anorexia, ending up bulimic. I mean I've never been bulimic, it's something I couldn't actually do. But girls that had been just starvers like me picking up about bulimia and ending up bulimic, which I thought was stupid. Anyway that's just my opinion about it.

I was in there eight months, and I'd begun to get really anxious to be with Matthew. In all that time it was almost as if he didn't exist, they never talked about him, I almost felt as if he'd been taken away. So in the end I discharged myself and I went home, but the problem was that nothing at home had changed had it? I was going back to exactly the same situation that I'd left, and I hadn't been treated to cope with home, I'd been treated in a very artificial situation. I mean the whole of the Falklands War had been and gone and I didn't even know, we were so insular in this little unit. My husband was angry with me by this time, really quite hostile, my son was eight months older and didn't really know anything about me, and I hadn't got anything else worked out to fill the void. I think it took me four months to lose three stone, all the weight I'd put on.

★ ★ ★

They didn't discharge me straight away. I went back after a month and the doctor looked me up and down and said, 'I can't speak to you if you've lost weight, I'm going to make it two months before I see you again'. So then I lost even more weight, and I rang him up and said, 'I'm sorry I can't stop losing weight', and he said, 'Well I can't see you if you've lost more weight'. That was the sum total of help I was getting.

I finally got back down to just under five stone, and I went back to see him for the final time. He looked at me, and he picked my hands up. They were awful, all crusty, broken and dry, and he looked at my hands and he said, 'You're in a poor way'. And I just said, 'Yes'. He said to me, 'I don't think you're going to last much longer. I think you are within a couple of days of death. I can't do anything for you', he said, 'I'm going to discharge you'. 'Oh, and by the way', he said, 'I should get in touch with your doctor if I were you'. And that was it. Discharged. That was it.

It was really quite good. Actually it was the best thing that could have happened in a funny sort of way. I drove home, and as I was driving home something inside of me snapped, you know – I thought, 'How dare he rubbish me' – I mean he'd let me go home to die, he didn't know how I was going to be. He'd literally said to me, 'Go home and die, you don't matter'. And I suppose you could see his point, I mean here was this woman, she couldn't hang it together, he didn't know me, why should he bother? So I drove home and sat there. Tom was away somewhere and I went into the kitchen and I ate a Mars bar. It was the first thing that I'd eaten on my own since I was 16. I always mark my recovery from anorexia from that day, eating that Mars bar. It really turned me round. Not that I started to eat marvellously and put on lots of weight straight away, I didn't. But I'd actually turned some sort of psychological corner inside me.

★   ★   ★

I managed to keep my weight stable at five-and-a-half stone for a year and a half, and bliss of all bliss I got a new psychiatric nurse and she persuaded my GP not to panic. He referred me to another psychiatrist locally, who saw me as having turned some sort of corner, and he said, 'You know, if you can keep the weight you are stable I won't interfere'. I don't think he knew what to do to be quite honest. The psychiatric nurse kept an eye on me and she became quite a good friend, she was really nice, very supportive. She might very well have been putting in the odd report to say I was fine and that Matthew was fine. So I can bless her for that.

I got into this habit of walking. I just used to set off in the morning, drop Matthew at school and walk, and walk, and walk, and walk and walk. I used to walk about 40 miles a day. It was as much to do with agitation from the drugs as anything else. I've got a vision of this terrible skinny woman wandering around Bracknell. I became the local freak, this skeleton strutting around. But it kept me sane, and as I walked I started to reason things out, and I began gradually, gradually to start increasing my weight.

I suppose I managed to get my weight up by a stone and a half on my own efforts, just doing this walking. It was a very good period for me, very slow, but I was doing it, nobody was making me do it, and I was doing it with the sort of food I could eat. I was actually eating extremely healthily. The thing that I didn't use to eat was carbohydrate and so I made myself eat carbohydrate at each meal. That was my medicine. And it was very therapeutic really.

★ ★ ★

But then I started to get a little bit agitated, and one day I had a screaming session in the street, and I was sectioned and put into St Bernard's in Ealing, a terrible old dump, I think it's closed now. And while I was there the psychiatrist had this policy of taking people off their medication to assess them, and I'd been due for an injection and I missed it. Then my psychiatric nurse managed to get the section overturned, and I was taken out of the hospital as she said she would look after me. My GP was on holiday, I'd missed my medication, and this was the major medication, the neuroleptics, and I had this incredible withdrawal where I went *completely* mad. I heard voices, saw visions, everything was all over the place. It went on for about a month or so.

I was so mad that I began to question all the beliefs that I'd had for years, and that I was part of some experiment began to seem really, really out of control. One day I turned to Tom and said, 'Would you stop fiddling with my brain? I can't stand it any more, just stop it!' And he looked at me, and said, 'What are you talking about – I'm not fiddling with your brain'. And it suddenly struck me that he might have a point, that there wasn't anything there. I couldn't believe it, my whole belief system fell away. I'd gone into a period of withdrawal from the drugs, and coming out of it everything suddenly seemed different.

So we had a great long discussion about all this and I got very upset. I felt utterly betrayed. Because everything that had happened to me I'd made sense of. All the unkind things and the cruel things, the way my parents had literally dumped me, and all those humiliating experiences in hospital, I'd turned them around so they were useful, so that I'd learned some lesson from them or they were good for me. I'd made it as if there was some point to them. Suddenly I realised that people had actually done all these dreadful things to me, and I felt awful, absolutely awful. I couldn't speak. I really couldn't understand the way I'd been treated. And I still didn't feel terribly well. That was when we came and found this place.

We moved in here and I started to hit a depression. I'd never been depressed. Here is a diary entry from around then:

I've never felt so dreadful as I do today, never felt so alone, never felt so terrified, never felt so utterly exhausted. I can no longer rely upon my escape routes. I've fought so hard and so long to come awake to this, this horrible awful life where no-one will understand or comfort me. My coping mechanisms have gone, I can no longer cope. I want to shut off my brain, it's all been too hard. Nobody can be that brave alone. Oh Christ I want to sleep forever now.

Life was black, I couldn't cope. I really thought I had come to the end.

★ ★ ★

I couldn't think what else I could do, so my husband called in a local psychiatrist. The irony was that this was the very first psychiatrist I had seen when I'd been 16, the help that my parents had rejected in the local hospital. He came to the house on a domiciliary visit and after I spoke a bit he said, 'I remember you, I remember you. You didn't want my help'. And I said, 'Well it wasn't me'. And he said to my husband that he didn't think I was schizophrenic at all, but he thought I was addicted to Mogadon, because I'd been taking Mogadon every night for 20-odd years, and that what was happening was that because I'd got completely tolerant of them, by the middle of the morning the next day I was going into withdrawal so that for the rest of the day I was getting hallucinations from withdrawal from Mogadon. And of course we just looked at him and thought he was completely gaga. I'd had 20-odd years of people saying that I was as mad as a hatter, and here he was saying that I was a junkie. And the funny thing was that I hadn't really rated this Mogadon as medication. I'd been taking these two sleeping pills every night, as I say for 20 years, and with all the other stuff I'd been taking they'd seemed like nothing, you know?

Anyhow I said to him that I would try and get off these things. He didn't tell me how. So I just stopped taking them, didn't I? I went cold turkey, and of course I was really ill and within about four days I had to take them again, I mean I had everything: the flu, the shakes, I felt really bad. So I went to my GP and he said, 'Oh you'd better take some Stelazine'. He didn't really know what to do. So I took this Stelazine; I only took it for about three weeks, and I thought, *this* is not the answer. So I stopped taking it, and I carried on like this for about a year. And then I began to feel so miserable that I wasn't making progress, I went back to the GP and I said, 'I'm going to come off this Mogadon, because I shall never know unless I've done it, and I can't feel any worse than I do anyway'. I'd got to the stage where I thought, 'Well I'm normal weight and this, that and the other, and life isn't worth living'. So he said, 'That's quite a good idea; cut it down just by a half, and have a go'. And so I said, 'All right I'll do that'. He was very good that GP. He's the best I've ever had.

So I cut it down, and within five weeks I was off it. It was quite hard, because each time I cut it down I had a couple of sleepless nights, but I was so determined to do it. I'd really got to the stage where I had no alternative left. When I went back to see him, his jaw dropped. He said, 'You haven't done it have you?' And I said, 'Yes'. Do you know, he did the nicest thing. He got up from behind the desk and he came out and he shook my hand. And he said, '*That's* amazing, *well done!*' And that made such a difference, I couldn't believe it. It really helped, that, because it was hell coming off those things. The symptoms for the next two years were quite horrendous, the physical withdrawal symptoms. Every symptom that you could actually get, I had. I mean, I was shaking, I got panic attacks, it felt as if my legs didn't exist, I had these terrible jelly legs, I was sick, I had flu symptoms, really, really awful. I didn't sleep *at all* for weeks and weeks and weeks. I started drawing then, and that was quite good.

★ ★ ★

About eight weeks after I started to cut down, I began to feel absolutely brilliant because my brain was starting to clear. I can remember waking up one morning and thinking, *I'm not mad.* It was a miracle really. I couldn't believe it, I began to actually feel alive. It was almost as if sanity started to creep in around the edges and the madness was dropping away; each day that went on I became more and more sane. I began to be able to speak without feeling as if my voice was coming from somewhere else, and one day something funny happened and I laughed, and it felt really strange. I mean I had not laughed properly at something for 20-odd years. Another time I was watching the telly and I felt something running down my face and I was crying at something I'd seen on the television, I'd been moved to the extent where something outside myself had actually triggered me to cry. I mean all my insides, my feelings were coming back. It was a complete miracle.

I just got better and better. My periods came back, I started to physically be okay, and the anorexia just disappeared overnight. I was literally eating normally without thinking. I stopped weighing myself just before I came off the tranquillisers and that was six years ago, and I haven't weighed myself since, and I'd been doing it 10 times a day. I no longer thought in any obsessive way about food. I have to exercise my imagination now to think what it was like to be anorectic. Things began to happen. I started to read and I couldn't stop reading, I read until my eyes fell out. Just to do things: to talk, to walk around the garden, go into town, just living, I was heady with it for a while. And the GP was marvellous. I used to go and see him, he'd say, 'What's happened? This is absolutely incredible'.

★ ★ ★

When I'd seen the local psychiatrist, he'd referred me to a psychologist for careers advice. And he was ever so nice. He sat and listened and the first thing he said was, 'I'm so sorry that we've done that to you'. I suppose for the last few years he's been debriefing me really. He allows me to go and see him every so often and I get 100 per cent support from him. He called in another very respected psychologist, and between them they've given me an outlet. Without having had those people to listen to me – who weren't involved – I might not have sorted myself out. I did need that debriefing. If I'd just come off the drugs and been left, I'd have got very depressed I think. Because ditching 20-odd years of your life you do tend to sit around and think, 'Well what the bloody hell do I do now?' And you try getting a job with a record like mine. Absolutely impossible – I can't get one. Psychiatrists tell you to lie. It makes me so angry that all they can offer their patients in terms of getting rid of stigma is to lie on a CV. It's shocking, absolutely shocking.

The first few months I was terrified because I thought I would wake up and it would all come back. I kept feeling the psychiatrist with the injection needle…it took me an awful long time to adjust. And my husband found it very difficult. I know he wanted me desperately to get well, obviously, but in the getting well there was a lot of pain for him. I think people who marry people or who live with people who've been a certain way, mentally ill or very repressed, marry that person for what that person is, and it came as a tremendous shock to my husband to realise that what was emerging was this woman who wasn't what he had imagined, somebody who was quite assertive and quite bright and did things and wanted things and lived. I found this made me very angry, because I was angry, I was furious at what had happened to me, and I think I was probably uncomfortable to live with. It's taken him a long while to accept me as the sort of person I now am. In many ways now I think we are probably the best of friends, we trust each other implicitly, and that has been worth fighting for, but certainly for the first year or two after I got better, it was very very difficult. I think either of us would have left at a minute's notice.

I'm very lucky in the fact that Tom can support me and enables me to do what I want to do. I tried to go back to university a couple of times, but it's not the right thing for me. I'm bored by it, to be quite honest. I went back and I did my Latin and Greek A-levels, and I walked them, they were a breeze. But when I went to the interview over at Oxford I thought, 'What am I doing here, this is so tedious, it's just not what I'm really about'. I don't want to spend all day stuffed in a library. I read Latin and Greek but I read it because I want to – and I read what I want.

★ ★ ★

Now I'm doing drawings and things and I've got plans. I had one exhibition which went down really well, and I've done a lot more since then. I actually went over to Ruskin College, Oxford, just to get an idea about whether it would be worth my applying to art college, and I had a long chat with the bloke there and he said that he thought it probably wouldn't be ideal because I'm self-taught, and people who are self-taught don't get on very well at art college because it's boring. You have to go at the pace of people who aren't interested and aren't motivated. But he said that he would offer me a place if I wanted. I felt ever so pleased – my head kind of expanded.

Just one last thing. I think doctors don't do nearly enough for people on tranquillisers. The fact that they still write the prescriptions, I think they should be struck off. They know what they do to people, they just can't be bothered to get people off, because it's hard. I don't think my GP really realised how horrendous it was. I mean I didn't have a psychological addiction to them at all, I knew that they were doing me no good, but it still didn't help. For a year afterwards I was craving them almost the whole time. I can remember him saying to me something like, 'At least I've got one person off tranquillisers'. And I said, 'What do you mean?' And he said, 'Well these people, they won't come off you know'. The trouble was that I'd been a success and he automatically thought that other people would find it so easy. But it's hard. That's the other thing – I used to go to the doctor at least once a week, and now I haven't been to the doctor for two years. Think of the money I've saved the NHS!

2.

Counselling was the turning point: Cheryl Stromeyer

A modern house in neat suburbia, manicured front lawn. It's not what I'd expected, but neither is Cheryl. A lively, middle-aged red-head, dressed in denims, she is very kind, going out of her way to make me feel welcome. 'Would you like some tea? There's some nuts and dried apricots here. Please help yourself.' Cheryl is an art therapist, and a natural care-giver. We sit in a large, open-plan room on beige velvet settees, overlooking a picture window onto the immaculate front lawns of the houses opposite. There's an overall impression of spaciousness and tranquillity, which is about to be disrupted by what she has to tell me. For years she was stuck in a very unhappy marriage and unable to see a way out. Her problems began when she was 29, after she had had her first child.

When I had my first baby I stopped working and moved to a completely new area with my husband. After having the baby I felt extremely low and depressed and tired, I didn't know anything about postnatal depression, all I knew is I should have been happy, there was something wrong. So I went to my doctor, and I remember very quietly saying, 'I'm very tired', and she sent me home with a box of tranquillisers. I didn't ask any questions in those days, I was a very passive person. I remember going home and my husband said, 'What are those?' I was quite frightened of him really, and I said, 'I've got these tranquillisers' and mumbled a bit, and he said 'You've not to take those, put them in the bin'. So I remember throwing them away and limping along for another couple of years and no-one, especially not my husband, saying, 'Well you can throw those away, but what is the matter, why you are feeling like this?'

★ ★ ★

A few years went by and I was very, very unhappy, that's the only way I can describe it. Then I had a second child, and that was okay. I was functioning very well. I was having in-laws here and making dinners and the children would be clean and well dressed and I was always on time. But a lot was going on inside which I was suppressing. I always felt I was doing something wrong, and my husband was a very critical man and had very, very high standards, so there was a lot of marital pressure but no outlet for it. I just kept thinking there was something wrong with me because it was my second marriage and if this was going wrong it must be my fault. And although I'd not done any psychology or psychotherapy I knew what my own childhood had been like: my father died very young, so I was from a family without a father, whereas the man I married came from a very stable family, a very conservative family, and he'd been sent off to public school. My natural way of expressing myself was really squashed by him, and that isn't now putting any blame on him, it was just that I was not assertive.

So I went back to my GP and saw an elderly doctor. I told him I was very unhappy in my marriage and I remember he said in a very quiet voice, 'I can send you to a psychiatrist or a marriage guidance counsellor', and I remember feeling very frightened. It was a reinforcement to me that there was something wrong with me because he'd linked a marriage guidance counsellor with a psychiatrist, and he'd made me feel it was my problem, he'd not suggested my husband came along. So I limped along again and didn't go to either, I didn't tell anyone. Oh, I fib. A friend told me that living next door to her was a psychiatrist, and I went secretively to see this psychiatrist and he was very nice. He said I should come back, but he didn't say I was mad; he reassured me I wasn't mad. I think that's maybe why I didn't go back; I'd got a verification, I suppose, and I just kept telling myself that the marriage would get better.

I must have gone to my doctor again, I can't exactly remember when, but I think I told my husband, and my husband phoned the doctor, and I think they were considering me as having some sort of mental illness, or brewing one, but those words were never mentioned. Anyway, a psychiatrist came to the house and I remember we had a very long settee and my husband was at one end and I was at the other, and he prescribed some medication. Now I don't know what it was but I took it, and it was a very frightening experience because it made me do something which I've seen people in hospital do, which is pace; I couldn't sit down. Every time I sat down I wanted to stand up, and every time I stood up I wanted to sit down. And I found myself wandering and pacing the house and I kept setting myself a task, thinking, 'I'll just defrost the freezer today', and opening and closing the door of the freezer. I didn't know anything about medication, I didn't connect the two in my mind, I just thought I was mad, this was what madness was. It was really terrible. It only lasted a week because at the end of the week my husband came in from work and I remember just crying and saying, 'I don't know what's going on,' and he phoned the psychiatrist, and the psychiatrist just coolly said, 'Tell her to stop taking them, it's probably too high a dose'.

★ ★ ★

I got it into my head that the best thing to do was to be more occupied, so as the children were toddlers, I didn't want to go back to work, I decided I'd do some work at a youth club. So I worked two nights a week, and for a while that really was the highlight of the week because I used to leave the house and feel very free, very relaxed, in contrast to how I felt at home. Then I read an advert in the paper that the Marriage Guidance Council wanted counsellors for training and I was interested in that. I went for an interview and they had eight prospective trainees together in a room, and you spent the day and had to do certain exercises. And at the end of the day I remember thinking, 'All the answers I gave were crazy', and then a few weeks later I got a letter of acceptance to say I could go for training and I was delighted. I remember my husband bought me a pen and said he was proud of me. And then I was given the name of my personal tutor for the marriage guidance counselling and something happened, something just clicked and I went completely. That's when I had an actual breakdown.

I'd taken the children to Sunday school classes at our synagogue, which they had to go to because they were going to have a bar mitzvah when they were 13. I was driving fine, and I was meant to go and visit my mother who lives out of town afterwards. Now in the synagogue there was a kitchen, and for some reason I just started to wipe the surfaces, it wasn't my job to do this, but I started to wipe these surfaces and everybody left except the Rabbi, and I do remember in my mind that it felt it was like the end of the world, and this Rabbi and I were going to start a new world with my children, but I wasn't sure about the children. I remember they had to come from an annexe and I went to get them, and when I saw them I was obviously in a highly emotional state because of what was going on in my mind, but nobody knew, and I thought, 'Oh, God has spared them', because I felt the rest of the world was going to be annihilated. I'd taken all my jewellery off. I had a diamond engagement ring, I'd taken it all off and put it in the dustbin, which again, nobody knew. I obviously looked okay, and I used the telephone. I phoned my mother and said, 'I shan't be coming today', and she said, 'Oh, that's all right'. Then the Rabbi said, 'Shouldn't you be going home?' And I said 'Yes', I remember putting the children in the car, but I couldn't go back to the house I lived in, that was what it was about really, trying to find a spiritual home where I could start again with my children, and without my husband.

I drove to the children's school, which was obviously closed. The headmaster there was a very nice, kindly man and he knew I was very unhappy, because sometimes when I took the children to school, if he said, 'How are you?' sympathetically, I used to burst into tears, and he used to make me a cup of tea and reassure me that hundreds of women had been in his room upset. Anyway I tried to get into the school and it was locked, so I got a brick and threw it through the window at the back of the school. I felt as if I was dying really, dying inside, and it was like a spiritual home…somewhere safe, where I was comfortable. Then because I couldn't get into the school I took the children home, and my husband looked very worried, I was about an hour late and he'd phoned the synagogue to find out where I was and they said they didn't know. When I walked in I said, 'I'm going to bed'. I was in a very strange state, and I just walked upstairs and went to bed, and he noticed I didn't have my ring on, which was strange. And he said, 'Where's your ring?' and I said, 'I put it in the dustbin'. And he phoned our GP, this time the third person at the practice came and… This is just amazing, because he just looked at me, didn't ask any questions, and just said 'You'll survive', I remember, or 'She'll survive', I think my husband was there, and walked out. So he didn't offer me anything, you know; it was an emergency call after a woman had put a brick through a window and thrown all her diamonds away and yet he just said, 'She'll survive'.

★ ★ ★

I woke up very early in the morning and very quietly got out of bed, dressed the children and presented myself at a friend's house at 8 o'clock, which was most unusual. She opened the door and I just said, 'Hello', as if it was normal, and she invited me in and said, 'Make yourself at home' or something, I mean she was a close friend, and I remember going upstairs in her house and just getting into her bed. The children were downstairs with her and she phoned my husband and he took them to school and then a whole operation was set into place. People came to her house, my doctor, my GP came, I was still in bed, and people kept coming to the door, and I remember shaking these people's hands, because in my mind I was someone very special at this point in time, I was a special person and they were coming to see me. So obviously the medical profession knew that I'd flipped, I wasn't behaving normally, and they decided among themselves that I had to go to hospital. And no-one actually mentioned that; all I knew was that people were coming to see me. Now to be sectioned you have to have two social workers, and I remember these two people talking to me and they must have known from their experience that I was in some other world. They said I could go somewhere where it was like home, and I remember going in a small ambulance to the local psychiatric hospital, but I didn't really know what was happening at the time. When I arrived there my friend's husband had brought this suitcase with clothes in and I had to go through these clothes. I have to say at that point I wasn't forced to take medication, and I didn't want to take any because of that previous experience I'd had, which was so traumatic.

★ ★ ★

Going into hospital was a really awful experience because I felt so abandoned. It transpired afterwards that not only was *I* not given information, but my husband wasn't given information, and he became very frightened and took the children away to his mother's in Brighton. They told him I was hypomanic and I think even the word schizophrenic was mentioned. And I think because they didn't give him any information he decided to get a second opinion, and they wouldn't let another psychiatrist come to me so all my records were sent to a psychiatrist in Manchester and I found out about this afterwards and felt very very angry. He did come to the hospital to say goodbye, and I cannot say I was terribly distressed about it all then, but when I came home and realised what he'd done I was very angry and distressed. So I was left in hospital and it was a horrible experience, really horrible. I wouldn't take medication, and they didn't force it upon me, but because I wasn't taking medication I was very high and very much in my own world and I wasn't sleeping or eating, and after about 10 days I was so desperate to sleep I asked if I could have a sleeping tablet and they said only if I took something else as well. I was desperate, so I said all right. What I took was lithium, and I got a few nights' sleep in and seemed to come back to normality very, very quickly, at which point they phoned my husband and told him to come and get his wife, which he did. I was only there for two weeks.

When I came home, I'd borrowed a lot of books from marriage guidance because that's what I thought I was going to do, and they'd all been squashed into this little box and put in the garage. And all the clothes that were in the wash basket of mine, that had been washed, he'd squashed them up in the wardrobe. He also had locked away my chequebook and credit cards, and he'd been round shops in the area asking people if I'd bought things. I think he was very ashamed. People afterwards told me that they had phoned up to ask how I was, because I was in hospital, and he'd said things like, 'She's all right but she can't have visitors'; he was stopping people seeing me. I think he found it very difficult to cope with.

I went back to work at the youth club after six weeks, but I felt so abandoned by my husband, I was so unhappy with him, that the breakdown made me say I wanted him to go, I didn't feel I could live with him anymore. And he said he'd go with me to marriage guidance counselling, so I thought I would give that a try. Obviously I had to abandon becoming a counsellor and they were very good and gave us an appointment. It was interesting because we went into this appointment and my husband sort of looked at the counsellor, beckoned to me and said 'I've come with my wife because she's got problems', and I remember the counsellor saying, 'There are three people in this room, and we're all going to work together with one sort of problem'. And I remember thinking that that gave me a lot of strength. It was only when I'd finished the counselling, I went for a year and six months, that the counsellor told me that when I'd first gone there I was quite incoherent – not mad, just not able to express myself clearly.

★ ★ ★

Once I'd had the breakdown my attitude to myself changed. I seemed to have a clearer mind, and I started to see that I wasn't mad and that there was nothing wrong with me, that it was 10 years of pressure and no outlet, and that was through the counselling. It was the counselling that really was the turning point for me, and one can only regret that I didn't have it earlier, but I didn't… It was a very, very important experience. We didn't go to counselling together, we blocked each other, so the counsellor suggested we went separately, and he found it very difficult. It made no difference to the marriage and eventually I decided that we needed to separate. I was 38 at the time. I don't know if I thought it was going to mean a divorce, I'm not sure. I was sort of battling for the marriage, but my husband very quickly said 'Put the house on the market', and divorce proceedings ensued. I think he had real problems with the marriage, but for eight years, the eight years where I was getting more distressed, more depressed and eventually had a complete breakdown, he was just going around as if life was normal and the marriage was okay when it was not at all; he couldn't have been happy within that marriage because there were definite signs that it wasn't a happy marriage. And although he would never have separated, he had an entirely different temperament and he could live that sort of second-rate life, and his first opportunity really, I think he took it. I think he could say well, I'd asked him to go, I'd made the decision, and he could think 'Well, it was my wife, she was an emotional woman and that was the reason for the breakdown'.

So I got divorced. I did a counselling course for a year and I started reassessing myself and seeing some of my strengths and that was very good. My marriage guidance counsellor had done some art therapy with me in the early stages; I was very blocked at one point and she said, 'Why don't you paint?' I'd been an art teacher previously and I had lost my confidence, so it wasn't something I really still owned, and I said 'No', but I was so desperate I did buy some paints and started painting and it was very important. Then a friend phoned me up one day and said she'd seen a creative counselling course, so I enquired about that and I went on this one-year art therapy course, a postgraduate diploma in art therapy – *while* I was bringing the children up here on my own. It was quite incredible: I was 40, so I'm going back nine years. I was the oldest person on the course, I had two children, they were 11 and 12, my ex-husband hadn't changed his attitudes about motherhood and he said he wouldn't help me, I had no right to go and do anything like that, my place was in the home looking after the children. Anyway I fought him on that one and he decided he would have the children one night a week while I stayed away for two days on this placement, which was part of the course.

When I was accepted it was like a new start really, so it was very important. I wanted to go without this label of mental health problems and the medication I was taking; I had been taking it about five years and I felt very flat on it, not depressed, but not right, and I felt I wanted this new start, so I stopped taking it. I went to see the psychiatrist who had prescribed it, and I said, 'How do I stop taking it?' and he said, 'You just stop', he said, 'You've got a 50/50 chance of this recurring, this hypomania', and I decided not to take it.

★ ★ ★

Now that year was a very stressful year for lots of reasons. I was doing like a full-time job because my placement was in a psychiatric hospital. I hadn't studied for years and years, so there was stress in the studying; my stepfather died during that year and he was in hospital for a long time and I was doing a lot of visiting; I was looking after two children and a dog by myself, because my ex-husband wouldn't even cook tea for them. And when I went off to my course Thursday mornings, I just kept my fingers crossed that all the arrangements I had made would come off. I had someone who came for the dog and took her for two days; I had the sitter who came in after school; I bought a microwave, the children cooked their own tea; I had my husband coming in at 7.00 collecting the children so that they could sleep with him, and I used to be away for two days just hoping everything had gone right, which it generally had. Only once did the boys phone me when the dog hadn't been collected and they didn't know what to do. I was very much on my own that year, I didn't go out at all, and towards the end I suppose the stress did tell on me. I needed a complete rest. I'd done my thesis, so I was right at the end, and I was at the college, very tearful, and I said to my friend, 'I'm going home'.

I came home and phoned my ex-husband up because I wanted someone to look after the children for a few days. But before he came round I'd gone to bed and I'd got a panicky feeling, and I put my dressing gown on and walked across the road to my neighbours, who I didn't know well, and I said, 'I don't feel very well', and they said, 'Come in, we'll make you a cup of tea'. I felt very unsettled and said, 'No, I'm okay'. I thought, 'I'll go outside and wait for my ex-husband', at which point he drove down the road and saw me in my dressing gown and that was enough for him to phone my GP. My GP came here, and I really can't remember what happened exactly. It was a trick really: all I know is that he took me to hospital and that was it. I was back in the same hospital for 10 days. They gave me lithium again and I came out feeling very, very depressed.

That experience was worse than the first time because I'd had a very big gap since the first time – seven years. I'd gone through a divorce, I'd re-trained, I'd been off the lithium a year. I think going back into hospital made me feel, 'Well, maybe this is going to happen every so many years, maybe I've got to take lithium'. I still wasn't able to see what I really needed, or to tell anyone what that past year had been like. And it was really odd: during the 10 days there was a weekend off, I was allowed out to my sister's, and my ex-husband took me back to the hospital and it was coming up to the time when it was my first son's bar mitzvah, and all he could talk about was the bar mitzvah and he'd have to have some help with it. It was very strange, my so-called mental illness never stopped my ex-husband leaning on me in some way, so I don't see it as a weakness, I suppose that's what I'm saying. Anyway, I got my diploma, but the 12 months after was very, very bad, maybe the worst 12 months of my life.

★ ★ ★

At the end of that next year I found work at a day-care centre for people who'd had mental health problems. The job itself was interesting because I'd been employed as a group therapist, but when I actually started to work there, I was in a team with two other people who had worked together for 10 years and these women had not had training in any sort of therapeutic work and I think they found it difficult to incorporate me, which made it very difficult to do anything therapeutic. I also found them to be very institutionalised and their view of the members concerned me, so I wasn't content with that job, it wasn't what I wanted. But I did it OK, and I carried on getting better.

Then I started to think about coming off the lithium. I'd read an article from *Open Mind* about a woman who had come off lithium, and it really inspired me. She wrote that she had very good friends and family and she spoke to them all and said she might have a weekend where she'd just retreat and come off the lithium. And I started to think about that and about my own temperament and about the things in life that were good for me and the sorts of people or situations that were not good for me, and I decided to come off the lithium, which was seven years ago. So I'm not on any medication, I'm not a patient anymore of anybody's, and that's felt very good.

I left the job at the day centre because this job came up which I've done for four years, as an advocacy worker for Mind, and it's been a very challenging, fascinating job. I've done newsletters, been to conferences, I do training of staff, all sorts of things. I wasn't employed to do anything for individuals, I was employed to get groups of people together who had mental health problems, because mental health services have changed over the last few years into community care, supposedly, and the area where I'm employed is undergoing change, and there have been lots of statutory meetings in health and social services where they've wanted users, and it was my job to get these people together to go to these meetings. That in itself was very difficult, because the people I've met have been ill. Now I don't normally use the word mental illness, and I don't mean ill as mentally ill, but they've been very worn down by the system, worn down by medication, worn down by no money, and they've not had the energy to get into that fighting situation.

★ ★ ★

Then about three years ago, something happened that made me realise that maybe for the rest of my life, I'm not safe from other people's perceptions of my behaviour. My mother, who's in her 80s and lives in a nursing home, had an accident and broke her hip, and it was through her having that accident that I learned that they'd been giving her psychotropic medication. I was still looking after my children, who by this time were into A-levels, I was still working, and I started visiting my mother. And she had an operation and when she came out of it there were lots of things that my sister and I were both not satisfied with at the hospital, and my sister said would I see someone about these issues. I asked to see the consultant and I was told okay, I was allowed to see him on the ward round. They'd given her this psychotropic medication in the home because they said she'd become aggressive and kept wanting to escape, but because she had a broken hip now she couldn't move, so I questioned why she was still having this medication after having had an anaesthetic as well, she's very frail and elderly. But I was told that that was the domain of the psychiatrist and this was the orthopaedic surgeon. I questioned a lot of things and it didn't go down very well I don't think. Anyway the decision was that my mother could go back to the nursing home the next day, which was quite a surprise I think to my sister, and I was delighted and so was she. And because it was such a long distance away from home, I stayed at my sister's that night, phoned my ex-husband, although the boys are well grown up and could look after themselves, I really just phoned him to say I wasn't going to be there that night and maybe they could all go out for a meal or something, and he asked me about my mother and I told him what I'd said to this consultant, and it was only in retrospect that I realised that when I told my sister, my brother-in-law and my niece, I remember there being a deathly silence. And I remember my ex-husband saying to me on the phone, 'calm down', which irritated me a bit, he was always telling me to calm down and why should I be calm [*laughing*]. I didn't actually think I wasn't calm.

I came back home feeling very very tired. My mother had been ill for three weeks, and I'd been visiting for three weeks and I wasn't sleeping well and I went to my GP and said, 'Could I have a week off work on compassionate leave and could I have some sleeping tablets for about a week?' She said,

'Fine'. That was on the Monday morning. Tuesday afternoon my sister arrived with my ex-sister-in-law, and they actually don't do much together and they don't normally visit me either, so it was very odd, and then the doorbell rang and my GP came in, so I had all these people in the room, and I got very frightened as I didn't know what was going on. My sister was saying she thought I wasn't well, and I remember feeling very angry, but I'd also learned through my job that the one thing a woman can't do is express anger. If you've had a mental health problem, you dare not raise your voice. So I knew I had to be very calm, but my sister looked angry because, she said, why didn't I take this lithium. My GP didn't put the pressure on, she just sat there, I think she didn't know what to do really. I was exhausted and went to bed. A very close friend visited and my sister I think told her to go, so there was a feeling around the house that somehow I was ill.

The next thing that transpired sounds like an exaggeration, but it's the truth. I'm in bed and about half past nine at night I got a phone call from my ex-husband to ask if I was okay. Now I don't see him often, and it was very odd to get a phone call offering help because my experience of him was that he didn't offer help. So he said, 'Are you all right?' and I said, 'Yes', and he said, 'Do you want me to come round?' and I said, 'No'. And then a little while after I heard a taxi outside, thought it was for next door, didn't hear the front door open, and my bedroom door opened and the ex-husband walked in. And I knew he had a drink problem, it's one that he'd always been able to contain, but had to watch, and I knew he'd been drinking and that for some reason he was over emotional. The next thing an emergency doctor walked in who I didn't know, and the next thing, a psychiatrist from the hospital where I worked. Then a social worker popped her head in, who I knew; I also knew that social workers only come when you're going to be sectioned. My sister arrived from the other side of the city with her husband, and this was all very late at night and I remember feeling absolutely petrified; I was so frightened. My children had actually gone to bed, and then I saw my son with clothes on, and what transpired was that my ex-husband had phoned here, told him to get dressed quietly because he said to him he didn't want him and Simon to see their mother being taken away. Now this is 17 years after the first time I was in hospital and I'd only been in hospital twice, once for 10 days and once for two weeks, which in terms of anyone's hospitalisation or time off work is so minimal, but it's so very major when it's in the mental health field.

I knew inside me that all I had to do was stay calm, it was funny, I mean there was a funny side to it. The psychiatrist said, 'How are you?' I said, 'I'm OK', I said, 'You know I work at your hospital, I'm the Advocacy Worker', and he said, 'Yes'. I said, 'You're very hard to get in the hospital'. And he says, 'Well just make an appointment to see me' – it was like that. I could hear people downstairs and I just knew to be calm, and they all left, but it was left that my eldest son was given a prescription for a tranquilliser called Melleril and he was told that he had to give it me. I still feel angry about this: I mean he was doing his A-levels, he didn't need that sort of anxiety and worry.

I took one tablet and it made me feel so ill I decided to put the lot in a plastic bag and take it all back to the chemist. Then I went to my doctor and asked her how had it happened that a psychiatrist had come to my house after I'd been to see her in the morning, how had it happened that all these people should descend upon my house. And she said, well she knew I wouldn't like this very much, but my ex-husband had phoned her, and she had acted upon it. So I went to my ex-husband and obviously had a dispute with him, and I told him that he was never to come to my house again and never to come into my bedroom again uninvited. I have a close friend who has agreed that if the doctor or anybody, a member of the family, ever think my behaviour is abnormal, she's the person to be contacted. She's a neighbour who sees me often and therefore if anyone needs an opinion her opinion is the most current one, and if I was ever stressed, she usually knows the reason and she knows it's just natural, usually something specific has happened, like my mother has had a major operation or something has popped up like that. So that's now left with my doctor, and it's agreed that my ex-husband has nothing to do with my life in that way. I could probably have taken the doctor to task on why she listened to other people and not to me. I could have really stirred things up. She knew I was angry, and I didn't know if I would ever heal that rift with my ex-husband, but what actually came out of it was that she asked me if I would find it beneficial to talk to a community psychiatric nurse, and an extremely nice man came here, and I went to him once, and talked about that night really, told him the whole history, and he said I was suffering from post-traumatic distress. For two nights I couldn't go into my bedroom, I slept downstairs, and my brother said I had to have someone stay here. My bedroom felt as if it had been invaded, it was horrible, horrible. I think the doctor knew she'd made a very bad decision, but in mental health that's what the supervision registers are about now, everyone else's fear is projected onto a person so they're a kind of a scapegoat.

★ ★ ★

This last year, because I knew it was my last year in this job, I thought it would be good to do advocacy work for individuals; go into ward rounds and go to their homes and really just support people, and I think maybe I've had more impact on the service doing that. But I'm leaving this job at the end of April. The funding was temporary and it comes to an end. I'm going to be working for myself as an art therapist. I feel that I've had such difficult times and it's something I want to do, so for my 50th birthday it's like a 12-month treat and if it doesn't work I'll look for a job. If it does I'd like to work in the Women's Centre in the city to start with, I'm going to rent a room one day a week. I can't afford to be a charity at the moment, but my aim is to take the art therapy to more people. I'm going to the Student's Union in March and doing a presentation on art therapy to see if any women there would want a group and if it could be funded, because students have very difficult times.

Therapy isn't for everyone, but it's certainly been my salvation. Being listened to at the age of 35 – just someone listening. What came out of all that therapy wasn't just about the marriage, it was also about my spiritual path and the difficulties of being what they call a holocaust survivor. I'm not a holocaust survivor in that I wasn't in Germany, and my parents weren't in Germany, but I was brought up as a child knowing that there was something not to know, which in my therapy actually came up as me feeling like a foreigner in England and trying to find my identity and my roots. In the art therapy I found, more than anything, it's your whole person that reveals itself, not little bits. And while I was doing all my training I did a year of the counselling, a year of art therapy without a qualification and then a year with, so that was three years' opportunity to be in groups and work through my own issues. These last few years also I've been going to an art therapy group – I think there's never an end, and maybe I'll never feel safe. But my life is always changing, so I see therapy as a most positive thing to do: it's about personal growth. I've gone through different processes, I've spent a lot of money on courses and weekends that I think are beneficial, where other people might spend their money in different ways. But I've had a firm belief from very early on that there isn't a thing called mental illness and I stay by that; I think it's the human predicament.

3

No easy answers: Keith Bright

It took me several months to get to see Keith. He'd happily talk to me for three-quarters of an hour on the phone, but he kept putting off meeting on the grounds of being too busy. Nevertheless, he would send newspaper cuttings, information he'd downloaded from the Internet, all sorts. I was on the brink of giving up on him when he changed his mind. I drove out to meet him at his house, in a pretty village in the Midlands, where he lived with his wife, Catherine. He turned out to be tall with greying hair, in his early forties. No sign of children or pets: on the contrary, their life seemed very self-contained. He had been made redundant from his work some three or four years ago and was still battling a tendency to obsessive thinking which had laid him low at the time. He and Catherine were now running a small publishing business from home.

I've been a journalist since 1980. We're both journalists. Catherine worked in a library for some years then she started writing for magazines. It wasn't really stretching her intelligence so when I got the biotechnology publication to edit I asked if she would like to be the deputy editor. She'd never done technical journalism before, though she's much better at interviewing than I am because I get really nervous. This doesn't scare me, to be honest. It did earlier on, but when I thought about it and we talked, the aims are very laudable.

My subject is biotechnology and genetic engineering; I wrote two reports last year on the biotech industry, studies that sell for about £350; you only sell a few hundred copies. I brought this through to show you. This was my first report on the biotech market. I produced it last year, quite proud of it really. When I wrote it I was in a pretty bad way, but it was therapeutic to do, certainly. At the time I knew very little about biotechnology because I'd covered life sciences before and I had to learn fast. There's a lot of interest out there in biotechnology.

I'm somebody who has always suffered from anxiety. At times it's been very acute, at other times it's been liveable with. But although things were difficult, for instance when I first went to university and when I was at school around O- and A-levels, I wouldn't say that I'd ever reached the point of complete and utter breakdown; I hate that word actually, but that's the only word I can think of. I did have a rough patch when I first started work in the early 80s, I had a trainee job which was very difficult, long hours, and I got really stressed by that. But things had really sorted themselves out and I was pretty well leading a normal life and almost put out of my mind that I'd ever had problems with anxiety in the past. Then I took a job in 1990, commissioning books on life sciences, and that was really when things started getting on top of me.

★ ★ ★

The division I was recruited for was relocating from Cambridge, and they didn't really want someone they had to relocate, so probably one of the reasons I was chosen is because I was local and the idea was that they paid for me to commute to Cambridge for however long it took. They said I'd only have to do it for about two or three months and then I could work from home and go up to Cambridge once a week, but this didn't happen. They also said the office move would be very short, three to six months; in fact it was nearly a year. So I had to work in Cambridge and for some reason I couldn't cope with that. Now I think probably I wouldn't enjoy it, but I'd put up with it, but at that time I got really worked up. It was also a very difficult job and the people I was working for seemed not to want me there; I think they'd wanted someone else and I'd been imposed on them, so there was a lot of friction, and it really got inside me. But instead of saying, 'Well, these people are the problem, the job's the problem, the commuting is the problem, perhaps I'd better get out and get another job as soon as possible, or give it a year', I didn't, I took it into myself and it made me physically quite ill in the sense that I was having panic attacks and terrible irritable bowel problems and sleeplessness. And then I started developing a problem which I'd had in the past, which is termed in psychiatric jargon obsessional compulsion or obsessive compulsive disorder. Repetitive worrying about some problem that just won't go away, and the more you think about it the worse it gets and the bigger it gets and the more out of proportion it gets and then of course the less contact it has with the real world. But whereas in the past it had been a pain and made life miserable for me, it had never been that bad.

It started out as work issues, with things to do with my expenses. I suppose expenses is a bit of a black art for most people in business. You try to be scrupulous, you try to keep the rules straight, but it's difficult, there are circumstances where you don't and most people don't worry about it, but I did. It got on top of me. I thought perhaps I would get found out by the auditors, trying to defraud the company, and of course I would get into severe trouble. In fact the amount of money we are talking about was probably no more than about four pounds. It wasn't even anything wrong, because when I eventually discussed it with people, they said, 'Well that's fair enough, that was your decision and it was a reasonable decision'. But it really weighed on me for a whole year, it got worse and worse. I had started taking the intermittent Valium when I first went to that company because my GP thought it might be helpful if things got too much, but it wasn't really helping. I mean you take a Valium and it lasts about half an hour and then you are left with the same problem. So I went back to the GP and said I had these obsessional anxieties. I'd actually started reading books on psychology to try and see what the problem was. It was really winding me up, because I'd be trying to do my job and I'd have all this nonsense. I realised at the time it was stupid, but it was a vicious circle, the more I worried about it the less effective I was with my job.

That GP was a young doctor, probably about 29, and he said, 'You've obviously got obsessive compulsive disorder. You'd better take clomipramine', which in those days was the drug they gave people who had that type of psychiatric problem. So I took it. But he didn't warn me that the side-effects would be fairly severe. I was just about to go on holiday, so on the week's holiday I didn't notice, I just felt a bit stoned. But then I went back to work and I was feeling terrible, couldn't drive; I don't know if you've ever taken those things, but they really make you feel weird, and it got worse. So I went back to the guy and he had the arrogance to say, 'You are obviously sick, if you like I'll sign you off for a couple of weeks so you can get over the side-effects'. But I said 'I can't do that, because it wouldn't exactly help my job'. So he said 'All right, I'll refer you to a consultant psychiatrist', and I didn't really think anything of it. I knew my wife wasn't very happy about it, but she didn't interfere.

★ ★ ★

I had real problems at work. It hadn't been going well since the early days and I felt so fed up, I thought the best thing that could happen was they'd sack me and I'd find another job. In fact after my trial period was over, they said, 'We're going to renew your probation for a month'. That was horrific, because although I'd thought they might fire me I hadn't seriously believed it, and being confronted with it was terrible, it really freaked me out. It was at that point when I first started taking Valium and sleeping pills and I must say it did help. In previous jobs I'd never ever had a problem. I'd always done very well. In fact I used to move fairly regularly, I used to stay somewhere for two years and then there wouldn't be any further opportunities, the job was boring, or not enough money, so I'd go elsewhere. But the problem was the recession came along and jobs were very hard to get.

I had quite a lot of responsibility in that job. I had about 30, 40 authors all writing textbooks for me. I had to make sure the manuscripts arrived on time and in reasonable shape and I had to liaise with the publisher and the publisher's deputy on issues such as publication policy, delivery, costs and budget, and with the production department and the sub-editors. So it was a job where you needed your wits about you. People said to me afterwards, 'Obviously you must have got ill because you couldn't cope with the pressure'. In fact the pressure wasn't the problem, the problem was that there were so many unknowns in that job, you just didn't know how many of those authors were actually going to write their books, a lot of them defaulted. I also had to travel a lot to get authors, and I didn't enjoy motorways, I used to get very panicky. The other real problem was my boss and his deputy. We just did not hit it off. They were perfectionists and very aggressive, and both having severe problems in their private lives and working incredibly long hours, which didn't help. They were very abrasive, and they just didn't know how to handle me. So whereas in my previous company the guy I'd worked with was very similar to me, he understood that I was something of a worrier and needed a lot of encouragement and a bit of advice and reassurance and you got a lot out of me, these people were not like that at all, they were very prone to panic themselves and they didn't want to solve problems, they'd throw things back at me. So I'd often not be understanding the job in the early days and I'd just be left in the deep end trying to sort it out.

★ ★ ★

So going back to the psychiatric side of things, as I said I started taking clomipramine, and I went and saw a psychiatrist, but it took a long time to get an appointment. By the time I saw the guy the side-effects had worn off and I'd got used to it, but the obsessive anxieties hadn't disappeared and what did he do, he put me on Prozac. I've talked to quite a few people who've taken Prozac and one or two say, 'That's a wonderful drug, it's solved all my problems', but most say, 'Yeah, it makes you feel very strange, it freaks you out', and that's what it did to me. And I'm sure at that point it became very noticeable at work that I was on some sort of medication. So I foolishly told people, I told my boss, told the personnel manager and I think from that time I was marked. And it got to the point with the Prozac that it was making me so panicky and anxious, it was just too much. So I went back to the psychiatrist after about two months of taking it, and he said, 'Oh well, let's try something else', and he put me on a type of tranquilliser which was higher class than Valium – Stelazine I think it was. Because I was so anxious by that point nothing could touch me, and he very quickly ramped it up from perhaps 2 mg per day to about 20, 25 mg a day. It was partly my fault, I would egg him on and ask for more.

After a while of this my body couldn't cope and I got ill, physically ill, my liver was playing up and I had to have three weeks' sick leave. I'm afraid that was the end of my job. I didn't actually lose it for another six months, but after that I think they were just waiting for me to be sufficiently *compos mentis* to give me my marching orders. So that was very unfortunate.

★ ★ ★

The psychiatrist had no real time for any sort of talking therapy, he was only interested in medication. In fact he had to take me off the Stelazine after about a month because it was obviously making me ill, but he put me on other things. And during the year that I was treated by this guy, he tried me on I don't know how many different types of tranquillisers and antidepressants, from haloperidol to flupenthixol to Stelazine to God knows what else. He had me on 600 mg of Melleril for about a month and all I could do was lie in bed; I had the maximum dose of haloperidol. I would try all these things and I'd feel great for a while, and then it would wear off, so he'd ramp it up. I suppose my mental state was getting worse and worse, I was getting more and more confused and anxious and the anxieties were getting more and more bizarre.

I saw a clinical psychologist for a while and I found him helpful to a point. He was a great one for strategies and he said something which I still adhere to, that if you have a plan for your working day, even if you are very anxious, you can always look at your plan and you'll know what to do. OK, if you're really anxious you can't do anything difficult, but you can do simple things like tidying up your office and if you go on with some simple things, in the end you'll probably calm down – that was helpful. What wasn't so helpful was he was a bit of a behaviourist. He used to get me to record an anxiety onto one of these five-minute looping tapes, and I'd have to listen to it. I would sit in my car at work in the lunch break, and my whole lunch break I'd be listening to this wretched recording. His theory apparently was that it would stimulate you to be very anxious at first, but if you did it often enough in the end listening to this obsessional anxiety would burn it out. I found it didn't happen; OK I might in the end give up on that one but I'd move onto something else.

At the very worst I would be quite tormented by my anxiety. I'd go to work and I'd be feeling very hot and bothered. I had a lot of hot flushes; in fact for me a symptom of anxiety is having a hot flush, face going very red. At that time I was getting rather paranoid about income tax, and I'd be worrying excessively about my income tax situation and I wouldn't be able to stop thinking about it. I'd probably phone Catherine four or five times during the day and I'd phone my counsellor, and probably the psychiatrist and the GP, and this was all in an open plan office by the way. And I'd talk to people at work, probably do very little work, especially once I was told I was leaving – there was basically nothing I could do, they told me just to tidy things up and get ready for someone to take over. So I just found myself sitting at this desk feeling very unhappy, very physically unwell and totally out of it, the absolute pits.

★ ★ ★

When things were really bad, before I lost my job, I foolishly went and talked to the personnel manager and told her that I felt suicidal. She was very unhelpful really. Actually I went to see her because I was looking for reassurance about an income tax issue, and she gave me the obvious answer which if I'd been in my right mind I would have known myself. But I started doubting: part of my problem was the fact that I'd seek reassurance from someone or check something myself, but then having reassured myself I'd doubt it and have to go back and check again, then I'd think of another reason why it wasn't the case. That really does drive one around the twist, I'm trying to think of an example. Well, the income tax thing, I rang the Inland Revenue about it and they said, 'Oh it's not a problem'. But I was thinking 'What if they start checking up on me, start looking at my tax affairs?' and so it would escalate and I'd keep wanting to check it. So I was probably spending all day at work thinking about this and seeing the personnel officer, and it was really distressing her because obviously she didn't know what to do with this guy who was out of his head, and I started telling her about the psychiatric treatment and about feeling suicidal and bursting into tears in her office, and at this point she actually lost her nerve and more or less said, 'You'd better not go out on any visits to authors, because we don't want you committing suicide in a company vehicle. I'll have to tell the managing director about you'. There was a lot of concern and obviously my job was at stake. And that really terrified me. It was a very silly thing to do; I mean in my right mind now I wouldn't breathe a word, because there is a terrible stigma attached to it. But in the end it became obvious because I was on such a high level of these tranquillisers that it affected my speech and co-ordination, I was half asleep almost. And my productivity, which had been very high, was drastically affected. I was working at half capacity and you can't get away with it in that sort of job. The problem was that the psychiatrist and the GP didn't seem to appreciate that while it might be appropriate for someone who's inside a hospital to get treated like that, give them lots of drugs and chop and change, for someone who's trying to hold down a demanding job, you just can't do it. They had no awareness of the reality, both guys seemed to think the drugs were the answer.

What really used to get me down was going to hospital to see the psychiatrist. It was a grotty hospital, badly maintained, and you'd see these sad looking people who were inpatients wandering around. The atmosphere in most of these mental hospitals is horrendous, there's this feeling of fear and despair, and it made me feel so much worse. So he'd see me and I'd be looking very agitated and he'd think things were really bad, and of course that would encourage him to over-prescribe. It was only when my wife started coming in the end and she said to him, 'Look he's not normally as bad as this when he's at home, it's only when he's here with you'. I'm glad I never actually went inside. I was tempted at one point, I asked if I could, and he said, 'No, you'll just have to rely on your wife'. It would have been the worst possible thing.

★ ★ ★

I think it was the end of August that year when I went to see my managing director, who said very simply that they were going to get rid of all the life sciences books and sell them to another publisher and my job would come to an end. Now I suspect that if I had been performing effectively that wouldn't have happened. They probably would have found me another job; there were other redundancies at the time and people were being re-employed at lower level capacities as desk editors or whatever. The fact was the books were not making a lot of money, there was a depression in publishing and a lot of competition from American publishers, but it was a terrible blow, no warning, and I was just beginning to get better at that point, so this made it 10 times worse. They gave me four months' notice, and I was out of work, effectively, for two and a half years. It was terrible really, because there weren't any jobs to go to, and even if there had been, I was in no fit state to start work. I'd lost so much confidence in myself and my ability to make decisions that I wasn't really fit to work for quite a while. The last time I saw the psychiatrist was just after I'd been made redundant. I'd been off clomipramine for six months and I'd been on amitriptyline and all sorts of other things and none of the stuff had worked. I was only on amitriptyline at that point, but I was on something like twice the maximum dose, and the psychiatrist had some blood tests done and they basically showed that this dose was too high for my metabolism. So he said, 'You'd better reduce it by half and we'd better put you back on clomipramine', and I thought, 'Oh no, this is ridiculous'. Even I could see at this point that this man was mucking around. I thought to myself, 'I'm not going to see this guy again, I don't want to take this stuff', so I came off it quite quickly, completely, threw it all away.

★ ★ ★

I found the withdrawal effects very, very difficult. I didn't sleep for three weeks, I couldn't sit still for three weeks – it was horrible, and then I started having almost psychotic, schizophrenic-type thoughts for about two months – that was horrendous. I've never had anything as bad as that since. Obviously my brain didn't like it, suddenly being deprived of some chemicals that it had had for a year and a half. I went through the works. I imagine that when people have the experience of dementia it was like what I went through: the brain was just firing off all this total crap and it was very scary.

I was still severely troubled with anxiety and obsessional anxiety. It didn't die down, and obviously having nothing to occupy myself with, it got considerably worse. But I was very disillusioned with the treatment I'd been getting, and also quite angry. Catherine was very disillusioned too. I think she'd been prepared initially to see whether there was anything to it. The psychiatrist was saying, 'There's something wrong with your brain, your brain doesn't work properly, and this medication will put it right'. They have a whole series of theories for obsessive compulsive disorder like they do for schizophrenia or manic depression. They seem to think that these problems are similar to epilepsy or other very obviously physical brain problems, and we'd fallen in with that for a while. But none of it had worked, the fact was that I had not responded to medication. The only thing that worked for me was high dosages of major tranquillisers, which is no good if you're trying to lead a useful, productive life, or live with people in a family. I suppose I also thought I wasn't going to get a job if I was so obviously drugged, because it affects your physical appearance, your eyes look sedated, your face looks drawn, and it gives you strange movements and affects your speech.

★ ★ ★

After I'd been on the dole for six months, I was called into the local Jobcentre and they asked if I'd like to go and work on a nature reserve with a load of other long-term unemployed. So I said, 'OK', I mean I didn't think it was going to help my career, but it was something to do. It was something called Employment Action, which is a scheme to get people off the dole, because you are technically employed when you're doing this, you get £10 a week plus your benefit. I only managed to cope with it for about three weeks, because the other people doing it were a weird bunch. It felt like a rehab unit – it was physically pleasant, but it wasn't much fun to be honest, working with people who had been out of work for 5 or 10 years, some of whom were also mentally slightly unbalanced. I was still applying for jobs all over the place. And then a job club was created for executives by a local charity, the Rotary. So this was quite a significant step for me, because twice a week I had to put on a jacket and tie and make sure I looked fairly presentable to go along to this meeting. It was a bit depressing because all these other people were out of work, but it was helpful because they were all positive about how they were going to get out of their situation, and what they were all saying was that they were not going to bother applying for jobs, they were going to go self-employed, which was a very sensible thing to do in fact. So after a year of unemployment, the penny finally dropped for me that I'd better try going into freelance journalism, freelance editing, and that's basically what I did.

I got some freelance work very quickly, but it was all intermittent. I might work for two weeks, then I would have no work for a month, so it was too risky to come off income support. The other thing I did which was helpful was I approached a couple of local publishers and said, 'Look, I know you can't offer me a job, but would you be interested in me doing some consultancy work for you on your book publishing programme, just for expenses and a fee if you get any books that are published?' And one of them took me on on that basis and I worked for them almost full time for about a year, from home. I produced a few books, but I was basically giving them advice on what sort of books to publish. I got about £1500 out of that and it was useful; it went on my CV and kept me busy. It was better than doing nothing. And little jobs like that led to other things. I got a lot of interviews, because it said on my CV working on a consultancy basis for these two publishers and people didn't realise that what it really meant was sitting in the spare bedroom in our old house at a primitive 286 computer, writing letters to people. They thought I was going into these companies' offices, so it looked impressive.

Another significant point for me came the following summer, when I inherited some money from a deceased relative. It wasn't a lot of money, but it meant that I could no longer stay on the dole because there's a threshold to how much money you're allowed to have in your bank account. So I came off the dole and that really forced me to be more serious about freelancing. But then the obsessional problems started up again, and I started mucking around with alternative remedies like magnesium. I don't know if you've heard this, but some people think that things like magnesium and other chemicals are good for anxiety. I wouldn't recommend it. I started taking vitamin B3, and magnesium and potassium, but unfortunately I started taking too much, like I had with the psychiatric drugs, and it was making me quite ill, so I went back to see a psychiatrist, who put me back on Stelazine and Melleril. The trouble was that I only saw this guy once and then I started seeing the GP, and I was basically dosing myself and deciding how much to take, which wasn't a good idea. I didn't realise then that part of the problem was that there was an element of me that was attracted to drugs, a bit like an alcoholic taking alcohol again, and had difficulty in controlling the drug intake. So after about a month of this Catherine took control; she basically devised a programme, which just shows that you don't have to be a doctor of psychiatry to help someone off drugs, and over two months we got me off them altogether and burned everything. This was early January last year, and I haven't taken anything since.

★ ★ ★

I suppose the way I am slowly but surely coming out of my black hole is through work. I am very fortunate in that regard because I am sure if I hadn't got any work, or been unwilling to go for self-employment, I'd probably still be in a very bad state. I was fortunate because I had some skills that were marketable, in the sense that I could edit manuscripts and write articles, and there is quite a lot of demand for journalists in the biotech field, so it was inevitable that I'd get some work in the end.

I started getting very busy with work last spring. Up to then it had been rather sporadic and not particularly interesting low level editorial work with the odd commission to do articles. Then I'd got what is called an Enterprise Allowance, which is a Government scheme where you got £1600 over 12 months in fortnightly payments. I didn't have a lot of work on at the time, but I had to put a business plan together and they gave me the grant and I also got a grant for buying a laser printer. That was a boost to my confidence. Before I published this report, I wrote one off my own bat about recent advances in genetic engineering technology, which I sold privately to a number of biotech companies; I earned about £1500 just doing that. Then about a year ago I got a contract to write another report, and I just had to force myself to say, 'Never mind what I feel, never mind what I'm thinking', I was still suffering a lot from obsessional anxieties, 'I'm just going to get on and do this work, because it's more important than anything really, working'. Not perhaps the be-all and end-all of life, but if you've been unemployed, the most important thing is getting back to work.

I still suffer a lot from anxiety. It's not as bad as it was, but sometimes it's very difficult. Sometimes the work calms you down, but other times you can't do it. So I have to be fairly flexible, and that's the beauty of working from home. For example, last week, I think it was Monday, I was getting very uptight, I just couldn't work, and I thought, 'I'll just go out in the garden', and I went out, had a smoke of my pipe and did a bit of gardening, and within about two hours I had calmed down and I was able to go back and do some more work. What was difficult in the early stages was that I'd never written one of these these reports before and it was quite a challenge, and looking back that was probably what was making me so anxious. But I just battled on, basically believing I could do it, and I succeeded, and they were very pleased. I did another one for another publisher. Then in August I landed this contract to edit a newsletter on biotechnology, and that was a great boost. I'd done a trial issue for the client, and they liked it and offered me the contract. It's good fun, very interesting work.

People say to me, 'It must be great, you're working again, you're getting reasonable money and you must be feeling great', and I want to say, 'No, I'm not, I feel terrible'. I keep panicking I won't be able to do it and I still have these wretched worries. I still find myself getting into these obsessive cycles of thinking about things. It's not tax and expenses anymore, last year I used to worry excessively about my racing bike and it was really getting on top of me. Aaah…I don't know. As I say, whenever it's manifested itself – I've had it going back, say, 20 years – it's always been in times of uncertainty and difficulty, and when things become more routine it's easier to manage. Of course starting a business, as anyone will say, is difficult; you have to work very long hours. But it's actually getting easier now because our publication is selling with quite a few subscribers, it's well past the difficult stage when you wonder whether it's going to make it. The reports I've published have done reasonably well, so I think it's going to be OK. I am hoping that as I get more used to work, perhaps in a year, two years, it will be just twinges, and perhaps in three years it'll be a thing of the past.

★ ★ ★

It's a pity it takes so long to recover. It's not like a physical illness where you break your leg and are back walking again within three months out of plaster. I think eventually it will pass away. I just get rather disappointed sometimes. Two sides to me, like a lot of people. There's a sensible side, a sensible Keith and then there is this silly barmy side that worries about friends and things like whether the cleaner will come in while we're away and help herself to our things. It really is stupid, but what can you do, life is too short. You just have to get on with your life in the end, try and live your life as positively as possible. And not allow yourself to have your life ruined by it. Get on with the work, try and get on with pleasant things, enjoyable things, and perhaps even on a chemical level, doing something pleasant actually stimulates the brain to work better.

Unfortunately there are no easy answers; there are no formulae: if you do this or do that, take this tablet or follow this set of strategies, you'll be OK. The only thing I've learned you can do with these things is to sit them out and eventually they go away. It is very distressing and you wish the hell it would stop, but it doesn't, it goes on for a few hours, even longer, and you just have to sweat it out. I think the alternative of taking tranquillisers can be helpful, but then again you could argue that anything which makes you relax, for instance having a swim or a bath or going for a walk or playing the piano, any of these things is going to help. In fact the best strategy the doctors used to tell me is distraction. So if you are prone, as I am, to worrying about something, distraction like work, or if that isn't helpful, reading a library book or watching the telly, is the best approach. The worst thing you can do is sit in a room worrying about your problem, trying to solve it. I've learned that if I've got into one of those thinking moods, no chance in hell of solving it by thinking about it. I just have to give it up and leave it alone.

4.

My music saved my life: Julie O'Connor

We met outside the mobile phone shop by the tube, the window and its phones dazzlingly bright on the dark winter's evening. Julie arrives on foot, leather jacketed, curly fair hair, big smile. I guess she's in her mid-30s. I'd seen her once before doing a gig – she's a performance artist – entertainer, singer and storyteller, and a disability rights activist. She is a natural comedian, telling jokes and stories all the way back to her flat about the condition of the Inner London boroughs, the government, the price of loo paper – you name it, she'll spin it. Back at her place she settles me down and asks a few questions about my credentials before telling her own tale. She has recently emerged from a breakdown following multiple bereavements and a lack of adequate support to help deal with them. Now she's in the process of putting her life back together.

I think my family background has a lot to do with the way I respond socially and emotionally to my circumstances now. I'm not going to get into debates about whether mental distress is caused by organic changes in the brain, physiological causes or whether it's entirely socially caused. I couldn't give a shit about those debates. Distress is distress, no matter how barking mad you are along the continuum, and I think these theories just divide and rule. I mention my family because I do think that's got a lot to do with it. I have two sisters with disabilities and I'm piggy in the middle of five, born between two sisters who died, a sister older than me and a sister younger than me. I think that had an enormous impact on me as a child. I carried the grief for a long, long time. I still feel I carry it, but that's another story.

I was first identified by the psychiatric services in 1979 when, as far as I was concerned, I was having a huge identity crisis. I went to my GP and just said I was very unhappy. A part of the reason was because I wanted to get out of university. I wanted to do art and drama and I'd chosen a technological university in Loughborough for fuck's sake. Anyway this GP had a good old look at me and said, 'What are your eating habits?' I'd actually lost a considerable amount of weight at that stage. A few months later I went back to the GP with some other problem and I'd put on an enormous amount of weight and she said, 'I think you've got an eating disorder'. And I said, 'No', but I was crippled with shame. I was sent off to see a shrink fairly quickly, and after that I flunked university, dropped out and moved to Trent Poly. That was a good move, apart from the round of psychiatrists.

I started off as an outpatient and I went from one clinic to another. I was transferred first of all to a woman psychiatrist who treated me like shit. I bumped into her in the street and she pretended she didn't know me, then the next week she wanted to carry on like I was a human being again. Bizarre. At the next clinic I was seen by a woman called Dr Lynn Dyer. I'll never forget it because when I got into the room the woman was over 20 stone and quite a lot shorter than me, very round and very angry looking, and I got these hideous fits of giggles, I couldn't stop. I took one look at her and thought, 'Well you're not fucking going to be able to help me, love, if I'm in here with an eating disorder − we're in this together in a big way.' And she said, 'What are you laughing at?' and I said, 'You', which was awful, but that was where I was at, and I couldn't stop laughing to tell her why. So she wrote me down for barking mad, she was just upset I think. She said that she couldn't work with me and she referred me on to another bloke, a psychiatrist, who I thought was a right prat. And he said he couldn't work with me and passed me on to some professor at yet another hospital, and then I started getting seen by a woman called Nuala Farrell. I saw her for about two years as an outpatient and she was brilliant actually: not that radical, but very loving and very human and prepared to take a lot of risks. There were times she would sit there in the sessions sobbing with me and I'd think 'Hang on, whose session is this?', but it was very human, very warm.

Well, I fell in love with Nuala Farrell, completely besotted with her, and when I realised she was going to be promoted I tried to kill myself. I'd been sent all this acid to sell by somebody who was a community psychiatric nurse, I kid you not, and I was very angry because this therapist had gone off and left me, complete infantile regression, and I took about 18 tabs of acid. I thought I was going to fly off the roof, just jump off the roof and die and that would be it. And no such thing. I actually became a cauliflower and crawled inside my brain and I was there for many weeks. I was well lost really and a bit out of touch with life for a while.

When I emerged out of that period of tripping off my face, I decided that what I needed to do was buy a camper van and fuck off and leave her to it. Not that she'd notice, but this was my theme, you know. At the same time I decided that the kind of therapy I'd had so far within psychiatry had made me very dependent, and I was very concerned that nobody should have that power over me again. So the day after I was discharged from St Margaret's Hospital, I started my training as a drama therapist. I didn't tell them I'd just been discharged; they wouldn't have taken me on.

★ ★ ★

Very solid training course, I enjoyed it. It involved being in individual therapy or analysis three times a week, group therapy within a training situation, and courses in psychiatry, psychology, drama and therapy – therapy being eclectic. So it was fascinating as well as equipping me with skills to ensure that nobody would do that to my head again, not without my say-so.

I decided to use drama therapy by dropping all the arty farty crap. I was using the group methods, the training and the underlying structure of the course to work in political ways where I could see fit. Like I set up a women's group for long-stay residents at a hospital for people who were then described as mentally sub-normal, believe it or not. This was only 1984; George Orwell was right. During that time, I started going wobbly again, felt very depressed. Part of it was that I just hadn't healed the wounds I originally had gone to pieces over. The kind of treatment I'd had only picked at the scabs. I didn't feel it had supported me or tried to find out who I was as a lesbian, or as a human being, so I felt quite distraught by a lot of it – really manipulated by some of the treatments, and sodden with other people's fanciful ideas of what normal is. The whole premise of psychiatry is white, male, middle class, heterosexual and able-bodied and I'm none of those, well I'm white, blonde-haired and blue-eyed in fact, but I'm certainly not heterosexual, I'm certainly not male, I'm certainly not able-bodied, and I just didn't fit the bill. I was treated for lesbianism for three years. Dr Lynn Dyer – she's the 'I'm so fat I can help you out of anything' – she wrote in my notes that I was suffering from a homosexual retreat. I don't like the idea that people can set off on their own creative writing exercises and scribble down anything fanciful about you from a three-minute meeting, which is usually the length of your time with a psychiatrist. If you meet with somebody for a 20-minute interview you're very lucky, that's an assessment, and even then they're sitting there with a list of tick boxes in their head: Are you depressed? Yes, No. Moved work? Yes, No. Employed? Yes, No. The whole premise is completely barking because you're not actually talking in human terms, you know: 'What do you see your difficulties are? What do you think brought you here? Why do you feel you're so distraught? *Do* you feel that you're distraught? Do *you* think you have a problem? Have you come here of your own volition? Have you been sent?' you know, and 'If *you* think there's no problem, why do you think *the doctor* perceives there's a problem? Let's have a talk about your relationship with your doctor'. None of that. They sit there with a tick list and, 'Let's look for the career case. One of these women one day will be my career case'. You can see it, the way they nod at you and the way they're casing you. But I'm too bright for that, I can dodge in and out of any bloody shrink who faces me, which has had its hard points because it's meant that it's been very hard to find somebody to work with who's been able to match me intellectually, to be able to really trust each other and talk about what's happening.

After training I got sent to St Albans Hospital. I got to the gates and looked around and I thought 'I don't want to step inside one of these institutions again, I really don't', so I turned away. I decided that whatever I did from then on, I would try and stay outside the system.

★ ★ ★

I got a job as a social worker, residential. This is hilarious. I got the job in the October, they sent a letter delighting in my success, how pleased they were to have me on board, invited me to the Christmas party in December. So I went to the party and I met with the staff and we made a work rota. I was due to start work on January 4th. January 4th came and a hand-delivered letter arrived saying 'We regret to inform you you were unsuccessful in your application, we wish you well in future applications for other jobs'. I thought, 'You fucking cowards'. I was furious. Then I thought, 'Actually, I haven't received this letter, I'm not taking it in'. So I went to work as planned, armed with the original letter, and I was told I had failed my medical. Well I hadn't been invited to a medical. In all the time I'd been at St Albans, I hadn't actually had a physical illness that meant I should go to a GP, but it was standard practice to provide on your application form details of your GP, and any history, and of course I'd given them to the GP I was registered with. What had happened was, standard procedure, social services had written and said 'We need a medical background on this woman'. This doctor who didn't know me looked in my file and wrote back, 'This woman is fundamentally emotionally unstable and unfit for work'. Nice innit? Dr Gillick his name was.

Jesus, I wiped the fucking floor with him. I went in and he said, 'What seems to be the matter?' And I said, 'You'. He said, 'I beg your pardon?' So I said, 'I have failed a job because of something you have written about me. So I need to know why you chose to do that because we haven't actually talked about this'. I said, 'If you have a new patient who you do not know and somebody writes to you and says can you advise me on this person's capacity for a job, why haven't you got the courage and the honesty to say, "I'll invite her in for a chat because I don't really know her"'. I said, 'You didn't do that. You didn't give me a moment of your time, nor the benefit of the doubt'. Anyway the long and the short of it was, I insisted on seeing my notes, I insisted that we sat and talked, and I insisted that he should correct the damage, and actually he was very good. We went through the notes together and I was outraged at some of the stuff I read, you know, sister's suicide attempts, social worker's intervention in the family from the age of 10 or whatever it was, and I ripped the lot up. I said, 'You can keep this' – it said chicken pox, German measles, glandular fever, allergic to penicillin – 'That's useful. This shit goes out in the bin', I said, 'And this', and I rolled some stuff up, 'goes in my pocket', and I put it in my pocket and the guy was shitting himself. I don't know what he thought I was going to do, other than he knew he'd been negligent and if I'd wanted to take it further I could have. So I took what notes I wanted out of there, but sadly I see they've been replaced since. All they do is they reconnect with whichever hospital it is and the notes are replaced from the computer print out. But at that time naively I thought I'd stolen my records and I was triumphant.

I got in contact with the then-called National Council for Civil Liberties and the Communist Party and the Labour Party and I went very public. I had nothing to lose. There was a spread in the local paper, 'Is This Woman Mad or Bad?' and a picture of me looking sullen underneath. One of the things I was saying is that these people are running a rehabilitation project paid for by public funds, you and me, the taxpayer. Now if they're saying I've failed the medical I didn't attend because I'm too fragile, I'm fundamentally emotionally unstable, then they're saying anybody who's been through the psychiatric system is not actually able to be rehabilitated, so what the fuck are they doing wasting all that public funding. So I scuppered them. It took me six months to fight it, but I finally got my job back at the end of July.

I was warned that my position would be very difficult if I tried to fight for back pay. Now I knew I was eligible for back pay, but I thought, 'This is a political decision, I've made my point here, I'm just going to eat humble pie', though we never really got on very well because I don't think I ever recovered from the insult. I told the whole staff team, they'd been given some complete tosh about me having cancer, and the team were right behind me, they were brilliant. So I worked there for a while and then I moved down to London, got a job with the GLC as a trainer with childcare workers. That was a hoot, had a great time. It lasted three months and then the GLC was abolished. Then I got a job with ILEA, the Inner London Education Authority, and of course that collapsed within a year, but because it was education I was taken on by the local education authority and I carried on working as a special educational needs lecturer in the arts in Camden.

★ ★ ★

I went into therapy privately, seeing alternative therapists, and didn't really get shunted back into the system for quite a while. I went to see this one woman who did body and massage therapy as well as talking therapy. I used to have a two-hour session with her, and we'd sit there and talk and get into really deep stuff together and then she'd go, 'Now take your clothes off and get on the couch' and I thought 'Aye aye'. God it was chaotic really, but I quite liked the anarchy of it and also I really fancied her so I went along with it. Then one day I went in there and we were getting into deep stuff about sexuality and violence and all this, and she says, 'We're not doing body work anymore'. I said 'What?' It's a bit like getting to see your lover and they say, 'We're not having it off anymore'. I said, 'We haven't discussed this'. She said, 'Well, I feel it's too intimate', and I said, 'Of course it is, it's been intimate for a whole year, for fuck's sake. Have you only just realised it's too intimate?' I was furious with her. I said, 'You cannot sit here for a year with somebody, they bring their most vulnerable self to you, you tell them to take their clothes off and then after a year you say, no put them back on I don't like what's happening'.

Anyway, she cried, which I was quite impressed with. She was very human. But I went back to see her because I was bloody furious. I went through this real grief afterwards. I said, 'You're a bastard', I just felt I needed to tell her. And she really touched me because she said, 'I'm so pleased you came back. I feel I made a lot of mistakes with you and I'm very, very sorry'. I was quite disarmed because I didn't expect her to come off her pedestal, I thought that was brave and I really took it to heart. I thought. 'Oh, she's only a human being, after all, it's just a bloody job'. So I shook her hand and went on my way.

★ ★ ★

This past four or five years I've had eight deaths, in really shocking circumstances. In fact the last one was just three months ago: my dad. That was less shocking because I always thought he'd die before me anyway, but it was still a shock. The first three were horrific, close friends, and I got very very depressed. I went to a Well Woman Clinic, I thought I was being right-on, I'd been for a smear test actually, as you do with a Well Woman Clinic, and I'd seen a poster on the wall. I said, 'I see you advertise bereavement counselling, I'd love some of that'. This doctor started to talk to me and she said, 'I really think you need psychiatric help'. So I said, 'Well, I am depressed, I'm aware of that, but I think it's a normal grief reaction, I've had three very shocking deaths, one of whom was a friend of mine I'd known for 13 years and alongside her bloke I nursed her through the end of her life, I was there when she died'. That didn't touch her. Anyway she gave me this letter to take to my GP and when I got outside the clinic, I opened it up. It said, 'This woman is profoundly depressed, suicidal and a potential risk, I think she should see a psychiatrist at once'. I was terrified. I went to see my GP and I said, 'I'm very sorry I opened this letter, but it really frightened me. I don't think I'm a suicide risk, but I do think I'm very depressed and I want bereavement counselling'. Anyway she didn't really know me, which didn't help, and she talked to me about psychotherapy, which didn't help. In the end she referred me to the local psychologist who gave me an assessment and said, 'I'll put you on the waiting list', which is what usually happens.

The next step was I was promoted at work. They were looking for a mental health system survivor to be their mental health coordinator for post-16 education and that was great, but the job was more stressful. I was supporting people who were tutors in adult education, specialists in their field, so they'd come as a photography tutor or a flower arranger, and they'd be thrown in hospital to run a group on the secure ward or the drug dependency unit, and it was just bizarre for them. I was there as their main port of call in a crisis and coordinator of support services. Another strand of my job was to raise the profile of mental health in education in the borough, and of mental health issues across the curriculum within the college [where I was based]. Then the last strand was in the area of psychiatric provision – getting people who'd been in hospital into education again and into living again. But of course no-one was helping me, and there came a point when I suddenly realised that the quality of what I had to give was gradually getting less and less, like I was shrivelling inside with grief.

I went to the doctor and I said, 'I really need help', and she had a few words with me and said, 'You're suffering from post-traumatic stress disorder'. I'd just had another friend die, fairly close to that appointment, and she sent me to see a psychiatric social worker who did an assessment with me and put in for funding, and I was offered a four-week stay at The Mill Crisis Centre. It was incredibly intense. We used to have 10 groups a week. We'd do three group meetings in which there were three shrinks in with the group, then we had art therapy, then dance or movement, three house meetings, and all sorts of fancy shenanigans. It was actually bloody useful, and I felt that I shifted an enormous load off my shoulders. I decided I wanted to go further with it and I went back for assessment and they offered me a three-month stay and said, 'We think you'd get a lot out of it', and I thought, 'I do too'.

By then I'd had six deaths; clocking 'em up. The first was a bloke I used to live with who was a really good mate of mine and the musical director of the theatre company I was working with. About a year after I'd moved out of the house he died very suddenly on stage; he'd had an aneurysm in his heart. The next was my dearest friend's nephew who was murdered, he was quite good mates with all of us so that was just awful. And then after that my friend Maz died of cervical cancer, she was only 28. When she first realised something was wrong nobody would believe her, in fact they put her on diazepam and told her she was hysterical, so she changed her doctor and on the strength of the notes her doctor upped her medication. In the end she took herself along to University College Hospital. They kept her in for the day, ran tests on her, and told her that she had the later stages of cancer. Her tumour was inoperable, but they tried to prolong her life; they gave her a catheter and an ileostomy – it was just horrific. By the end she had gangrene in both legs, the tumour was visible on her arse, and she had kidney failure, heart failure, everything. Awful.

After Maz, Jean died. She was the woman who used to run the pub where we did music sessions every Tuesday, and that was a bloody shock because she'd decided to leave the pub, so we'd gone to give her a farewell concert. Two weeks later she stepped off the curb and somebody ran her over, hit and run.

Then Nicki died a year ago. She'd been knocking around with us for years, me mate's partner, left a baby of seven months behind. She drowned in peculiar circumstances, and that was a bloody shock. Then straight after that my uncle died, which was peculiar because he was a fit, funny man. Then a woman I worked with in the summer months was run over just up the road, she was knocked down by a 12-tonne truck, which was horrific. Anyway, throughout this time I was prescribed various medication. Then I went in for my second stay at The Mill.

★ ★ ★

If I'd trusted my guts I would have turned around on day one and come home, because something didn't feel safe there. When I was there first of all there was a group of resident therapists who knew each other very well, they were a strong team and they'd been working there for some time. This time the team felt very fragile; two of the members had only been in post six weeks; both were very young, one of them was only 26, and that made for a *very* different environment. The two people who were younger than me weren't as well trained as I am, for God's sake. One of them was a psychiatric nurse it has to be said, but she was actually very distressed herself, and I was in a great deal of distress at the time. My sister just older than me who has spina bifida was going through a huge crisis. She'd been in a lot of pain and difficulty with an infection in the leg bone that had spread to her hips. She was told that she might have to have part of her foot amputated, and she was terrified. They managed to get rid of the infection by putting her on a penicillin drip, but then she suddenly flipped out and went to Spain, leaving the kids behind and everything. The result of all this was that she lost custody of the kids, which was awful. So I was struggling with the grief of that, never mind all the other stuff I was trying to sort through: why all these people were dying, had I caused it? I felt like I was a hex in the world.

I had spent three and a half weeks of my three months in The Mill, all paid for, and on the last morning we had an art therapy session that went horribly wrong. There was a very vulnerable young boy in there, a survivor of satanic ritual abuse (though I'm not sure he survived actually), and I befriended him. He was very much on the edge. On the day in question he slashed his wrist and the art therapist went home in distress. She described the session as 'desperate'. One therapist had gone away on holiday, and this very young nurse was on duty, wet behind the ears, straight out of psychiatric nursing. She went out shopping for food – 'just to get out of the therapeutic milieu', she said – and a trainee therapist called Kevin was transported in to look after us, he was a baby sitter really. I can only tell you what I can remember of what happened next, because much of it is very fragmented.

I was feeling very distressed. I was really worried about this guy who'd gone off and slashed his wrist and been bandaged up. I'd gone upstairs to my bedroom, and there was a knock on the door and he came in with his cutter and said, 'Hide it for me, I don't want to do it again'. I thought that was a really trusting thing to do, so I hid his cutter and he said, 'Please come downstairs, I want to talk to you'. So I went down into the living room where this trainee therapist Kevin was. Now he'd gone out with this guy who'd just been bandaged up, and brought back two horror movies. Now can you believe colluding with this, even if the young guy had chosen them himself? One of them was about some carnivorous devil that ate children and the other was about a young bloke – Lawnmower Man, or something – who becomes some kind of demonic super power that takes over the world. Oh, and a bottle of tonic wine.

I queried the choice of films. Nothing was said, so I sat down and was talking to this guy who'd just been bandaged up and then there was a knock on the door. Kevin went to answer it and he let these people in, three local senior clinical psychologists who'd decided to drop by. It felt very much like they'd come to see the monkeys, very intrusive. Anyway he started showing them around and he was talking about us, saying, 'Of course these people would be in hospital if it wasn't for us, blah, blah'. I thought, 'You smug, arrogant little prat'. So I decided to put my mental health role on, I stood up and said, 'Gentlemen, thank you so much for calling, but it is rather an inconvenient time, and we'd prefer it if you'd make an appointment. Do call again, thank you'. I just stood there with my arms folded, warmly thanking them. They went, 'Yes, of course, sorry', and left. And he stood there, Kevin, the trainee, knob-head, 'Oh that frightened them didn't it?' And I said, 'No Kevin, that frightened you, do it in private next time'. I was insulted, I felt invaded, and I thought he'd been completely unprofessional letting those people in at that point, given the house was so fragile and that people felt so desperate, desperate enough for the art therapist to go home in distress. Anyway, bad judgement on my part, but I sat down drinking with them and I didn't check what was in the bottle. Then I went downstairs into the cellar and got another bottle of red wine, and my flesh started creeping and crawling and I started to buzz. I was starting to feel really aggressive and everyone was moving really slowly, it was annoying me they were so slow. I thought 'Speeding? Why am I speeding?' I went into the kitchen and I said, 'I think something's happening to me'. I was all shaky and Sue looked at me and she said, 'Your eyes look wild, what's happened?' I said, 'I think I'm gonna blow'. I went back into the other room and had a look at the bottle and I thought, 'Oh fuck it's caffeine'; I'm completely hyper on caffeine and I really avoid it.

★ ★ ★

I suppose it was toxic shock, coupled with the anger of my response to this guy and the way he'd behaved as a trainee therapist, supposedly caring for us and supposedly in charge, but I completely blew. I'm told I put my head through every window in the downstairs of that building, I'm told that I head butted him and kicked him in the groin and sent him flying through the door, I'm told I terrified the life out of anybody who got in my way, and I'm told that I completely destroyed the consult office in the back of the building. Well the only things I actually remember that evening are going into the kitchen and going, 'I think I'm going to blow. Can somebody help me?' I remember hitting my head on something and then seeing all this cracked glass and lots of light through it and thinking 'My, how beautiful the light looks through there', and then I remember somebody screaming, it could have been me actually. Then I remember being dragged out of a bush by six police officers beating the shite out of me, and then something on my ankles, handcuffs behind my back and being thrown on my belly into a van. I remember a foot behind my neck and a foot on my back so I couldn't move, and people telling me to 'Shut the fuck up', and then I remember having my shoes and half my clothes removed and being thrown in a cell. And from then on everything is very clear because it was so shocking.

★ ★ ★

I can remember the cell, I can remember the smell of piss, I can remember it was a blue blanket that needed darning, I can remember how high up the window was, it had six bars, I can remember turning round and seeing that there was no toilet but there was a little silver can thing with a lid, I can remember turning back and looking at the door that they'd just closed behind me and there was a hatch with three bars, and you could pull the hatch back, but only from their side, and there was a buzzer by it. So I *kept* my finger on the buzzer until somebody came and I said, 'I'm allowed a phone call, I know my rights'. And they said, 'No you're not, you're mad', and shut the door. They must have taken me in about 7 o'clock, and I was kept 'til about midnight, one o'clock, maybe, and then I was frog-marched outside and they gave me my jumper back and threw my shoes at me and said, 'Sign for your things.'

They handcuffed me again and took me on my belly again in the back of the van. I'll never forget, I couldn't get the smell of piss out of my nose, they'd obviously had somebody in there who wasn't continent. They took me to the lock-in at St Margaret's. I only knew it was St Margaret's because when they marched me out of the van I could see the sign on the side, and I knew it was the lock-in because the doors all lock as you go in – there's this terrible sensation of layers and layers of locked doors behind you. So the first thing I wanted to do was go to the toilet, I was in panic. I said, 'I need to go to the toilet', they said, 'No you can't, mate'. Now admittedly there were only three officers with me accompanying me on the way back; on the way there were six officers who beat me up. Caring, isn't it?! At no time was I ever accompanied by anybody who was trained in mental health. And what is very sad in the whole story is that nobody at any time actually explained to me what was happening, explained to me that I'd gone off my trolley and become very distressed and smashed the place up and people were frightened. Once inside the hospital I was in a complete state of shock, I mean I was treated for the shock for months afterwards. I was covered in bruises. I had the mark of a black jackboot on my back. I had bracelet marks up and down my wrists where the handcuffs were too tight. I had bruises on my ankles, and I had a huge bruise on my forehead which is where I must have been butting the windows or whatever the fuck I'd been doing.

What I then remember is coming to very quickly and realising 'I've got to play my cards right here'. It's amazing how quickly you can sober up, literally. The two doctors in attendance were trying to put me on a section 74 or a 4, which is risk of self-injury, and they couldn't because I looked at them and I said, 'This is an improperly applied section, you won't get this to stick, and furthermore you don't have a psychiatric social worker present.' And one of these guys looked at me and said, 'How do you know so much?' I said, 'I'm mental health coordinator for Camden education', and he just laughed and said, 'Oh yes, what's your name, darling?' I told him my name and I said, 'You can verify that when you check the payroll'. And then of course they played games with me, 'How do we know you are who you say you are?' And I said, 'Well truly, without my cooperation, you don't know you're born'. I said, 'Let's not play games, I know who I am'. So then he said to me 'I don't think you're mentally ill at all, I think you're criminally insane'. So I said, 'Well that's your choice'. Then I said, 'I suggest you remove the handcuffs because

I'm already on a lock-in ward, I'm already effectively detained and this is illegal also'. So one looked at the other and then they looked at the cop and they went next door, and there was an almighty row. 'No I'm not fucking arresting her, she hasn't done fucking nothing wrong, I'm not. You asked me for the fucking paper work, you wanted a 136, you've got a fucking 136, you do the rest of it.' And they're going, 'Well we can't section her, we think she's a criminal'. I thought 'Just play your cards right and you'll get out'. Well I was released, they couldn't apply the section, and thank God.

The next morning I was released, but I had to sign a piece of paper saying I was going with the police of my own volition. I'm not sure what the hell I signed. I was just convinced that if I didn't sign this I'd get a needle up the bum, and that maybe months later I would re-emerge out of the cloud of fog and perhaps never have my life back again. As it is, my life as it was then was completely destroyed, because by the next day my line manager had rung up from work, just by chance, to find out about a piece of work that I'd delegated. She was informed over the phone that I'd been sectioned and she could find me in St Margaret's, which was completely confidential and actually wasn't accurate. She took that back to her director, who asked questions; the rumour then circulated that I'd attacked a therapist and that I was now a danger to the public. So my case was then sent to an external occupational health team for assessment and I was called in to see a Dr Mcsomething in the next borough just a couple of months later, and it was impossible to ever return to my job. Shortly after that I lost my home, which was part of my other job – I was living in a community for people with learning disabilities, and I got the flat in exchange for social work, and I couldn't sustain the role anymore. I'd lost a lot of courage and a lot of strength.

★ ★ ★

First of all I kept my head down. I have to say that my partner at the time was really supportive. She came the next day with flowers to see me at the centre, and it was all boarded up and she couldn't understand why. They came to the door and said that I wasn't there, and she said, 'Well, where is she?' They said, 'Well you might find her at the hospital or if she's not there she might be at home'. They were really cagey. And she said, 'Hang on, I'm her next of kin, we've been together nine years'. Anyway she found me at home, so paranoid I was just cowering in the corner. I was convinced the police were coming back and they'd find me, and I was covered in bruises. I was so raw I couldn't really cope with human contact. So she got me out of there, she said, 'Come on, you're coming home with me'. And I stayed in hiding really, a virtual recluse at her house for four weeks, during which time I struggled to make sense of what happened. I wasn't allowed near the centre; they told me if I came near the centre I had to be handcuffed to an officer at all times. They'd kept all my things, I didn't get my clothes back for eight days. I wasn't allowed to see the therapist who I'd seen for six months, three times a week. She refused to work with me. I wasn't allowed to see the people who were present on that day, and I wanted people to tell me what had happened. I could only piece together what I remembered. The young boy who'd been so badly hurt kept ringing me up and saying, 'I'm going to fucking kill those bitches, they've stitched you up', and I thought, 'Well who? Who stitched me up? Why?' So he was left with all sorts of dangerous stories going round in his head as well.

It went from bad to worse. This hospital transferred me to Camden Hospital. The psychiatrist who had tried to section me, the one that ended up in a fight with the police, was supposed to send a clinical report to Camden Hospital, it was never sent. He was also supposed to send a clinical opinion with The Mill's clinical assessment because he was the consultant psychiatrist attached to The Mill Association. Well neither of them ever got it together, so when I was finally given an appointment three months later, in a terrible state I have to say, profoundly shocked and traumatised, the doctor I saw said, 'I can't see you because I don't know anything about you. All I have is your name and none of your notes have arrived'. I went fucking nuts.

After that I was on serious levels of medication, and then they decided to send me for brain scans and EEGs: they decided I was brain damaged. So what they did was they ran these scans and they proved that I'm hyperactive. Great, any of my mates could have told them that, I could have told them that myself. Waste of bloody money, 400 quid a time for a brain scan, God knows how much for EEGs. And they called back and said they wanted me to come back a second time because there were marked spiked motions on the right side of my brain and they wanted me to go under a sleeping draught and I thought 'Right brain, right hemisphere, creative'. Most of my life has run round creativity, I'm a musician, for fuck's sake, I'm a playwright and a writer, that's what I do. I sleep, eat, dream, creative arts, always have done, that's my passion, and they are talking about medicating me so there's no personality left – fuck that. They wanted to give me something that calmed down the right hemisphere spiking, I thought, 'That's probably my personality. What are we talking about here?' So I said, 'It doesn't worry me that my right hemisphere spikes, does it worry you?' The shrink at the time said, 'Well, it might be that you have a susceptibility to epilepsy'. And I said, 'Well I think I'd have noticed, and if it ever happens I'll come back to you, or I'll paint a picture, or I'll talk about it to somebody, but I'm not going to take any drugs'.

So I'm thrown back in the world. I'm supposed to be still on medication, it has to be said I've weaned myself off and I self-medicate. I drink wine if I think I need to sleep, and occasionally I use sleeping tablets, but I use them when I want to, not when they dictate. I went back to my doctor last week and I said, 'This may sound eccentric, but two years ago I asked for bereavement counselling. Now I wonder, I've been a dutiful daughter for two years, I've taken the medication, I have been in the hospital, I went to the clinic and out again, I have had two brain scans, I have also had two tests of EEG, now do you think you could just give me the bereavement counselling?' And she looked at me and said, 'Do you mean you never actually had bereavement counselling?' I said 'No, you sent me to see a shrink, who sent me to see a shrink, who sent me to see a shrink'. Which is absolutely the truth. The last one finally sent me to see a woman psychiatrist at Barts, I used to call it Barks. I was there for six months with this woman to 'get to know each other'. Bereavement counselling – no. I kid you not. That was supposed to be holding therapy to talk about my traumatic episode at The Mill. And I keep saying, 'But my dad's just died, but, but, my dad's just died, do you think somebody somewhere could offer me some bereavement counselling?' I think I know what I need. It's a pity they don't.

★ ★ ★

I think my music saved my life, I really do. Going back to that first suicide attempt when I took loads of acid, and instead of leaping off the roof I went right inside my head and thought I was walking round a cauliflower. I kept having images of being scattered to the four corners of the earth; it was a really spiritual experience. I could hear music from every corner of the earth, and I felt like every cell of my body had its own tone and its own harmonic. When I emerged out of this complete trip I was singing all the time, caoining my grief and singing sad songs. And I went back to my roots because one of the things that stayed with me was the sense of every cell of my body being full of ancient memory, and that the songs and stories were important. So I went back to Ireland gathering songs and stories and became obsessed with the Sean Bhain Bhocht, the Old Woman of Ireland, who is Ireland itself, caoining her grief away and continually shedding tears in order to replenish the land and refertilise the soil ready for growth. I loved that image.

I'm really interested in this woman's work I've just heard about, Sharee Edwards. She does this thing called Sound Signature. She believes that every one of us has various sounds throughout every cell of our body and sometimes there are certain sounds missing, and she only needs to hear your voice and she can pick out the sound that you're missing and sing it to you; it's part of her healing. Actually I'm thinking of doing her training. I like the idea of moving forward into something more spiritual with voice that picks up on that idea of having sound in every cell of your body. It beats the shite out of Prozac, I'll tell you.

You saw the cabaret show I did. I do loads of that. I did four weeks in Greece, came back, was here two days, and after that I was in Ireland helping to launch an album which I'd produced. We were recording and I was performing there, and I was the compere as well for the tape launch, which was on RTE television and radio. Came back, I was in Leicester at the Y Theatre and the next day I was in Birmingham, Midland Arts Centre, back in Leicester at the YMCA. After that I was up in Blackpool, then down in Manchester, and then this week I'm up in Liverpool for two gigs, so it's quite a lot of work performing-wise. If I wasn't so lazy I'd have a lot more work. I'm not good at self-promotion, like I haven't done any leaflets. But I did manage to finish this tape. I must give you a copy, then you'll get an idea of the old caoining, wailing woman of Ireland.

What I tend to do is stories and poems and songs that fit in. I've got a piece called *Through the Eye of the Storm*. That's my main focus at the moment. It's about literally going to hell and coming back, and the stillness in the chaos at the centre of the storm. There's always a place of absolute stillness, which it takes enormous courage to go to and sit in and sit with, because you have to trust that you'll be able to come out the other side.

PART TWO

Women survivors of childhood abuse

5.

I was lucky in a way:
Steph Corby

We met at the central station. Steph is in her mid-20s, with a curly mane of dark hair, tied back in a pony tail. She had dressed up in a tartan suit. 'My husband's dead jealous, he thinks I'm seeing another man', she said. We stopped for coffee before heading back to their place, a starter unit on an estate a couple of miles out of town. She showed me round, talking all the while about her husband, Garth, their two kittens, the new house and the souvenirs from around the world that covered the walls and shelves. 'Garth brought these back from when he was on his travels – he used to be in the army.' Steph and her husband are both mental health service users; he since the army, she since her schooldays. She has a history of self-harming behaviours.

I didn't have a very happy childhood. My mum was very verbally abusive as well as physically abusive, and I was sexually abused by my father from being a very young girl. It's one of the reasons my parents split up, I think, because my mother found out. My mum and dad split up when I was eight, so it was some years before that. I don't really remember. I've had flashes in counselling, but I never knew that I was being abused until about a year ago because I used to be able to blank things out.

All the way through my school years I never got on very well. We moved up North from Suffolk where my father was working at the RAF base because my mother and father got divorced. It was quite a rough school where I went to junior school, then I went to quite a posh school. So I was ridiculed in the first for being too posh and in the second one for not being posh enough. And everyone used to make fun of me because I was a bit of an ugly duckling. My mum was playing the abuse on me – she made me look bad, gave me a terrible haircut, she made me wear terrible clothes – I was a laughing stock really.

Everybody was matching me up with the most undesirable males going and making jokes, things like that.

I suffered from paralysing migraines from when I was 15, which meant I had to take an awful lot of time off school. I didn't actually do any work for my GCSEs until about three weeks before – I didn't even have a textbook for some of the lessons – I just blagged my way through. I did my GCSEs, got some really good grades, and decided to go to the sixth form. I took maths, further maths, physics and French. I was working at the same time after hours at a local fish factory.

★ ★ ★

I first came into contact with the mental health system when I was in the sixth form. Things had been going very badly. I wasn't doing the work, I wasn't feeling well, I was having a real bad time, and with all these problems I started to drink a bit as well. I was drinking vodka and orange a lot when I was in the sixth form. Then I had a long-distance boyfriend, but he found somebody else and I took my first overdose when I was 16. I took 50 paracetamol without even knowing what I was doing. I was at work at the time and half an hour later I thought, 'I don't feel poorly. I don't feel like I'm going to fall over', so I went to try and take some more. But because of the paracetamol my tummy reacted, my throat closed up, and when I tried to swallow some more tablets I just threw the rest up. After that I tried again with some migraine tablets my doctor had given me. We were supposed to be doing this project, me and these two other girls. We went down to the lab to see a teacher who was helping us out, and they both started on me, and I just completely snapped and yelled at them. I left my bag and ran out of school all the way down to a telephone box, and I phoned my boyfriend, who was a different boyfriend by then. My boyfriend suggested that I go to see the Samaritans. So I went to the Samaritans, and they called in the supervisor because I was still a minor, and the supervisor managed to get me my first psychiatric outpatient's appointment. I only ever saw this psychiatrist twice because it was so depressing. The last time I saw him I went out and overdosed afterwards because I was feeling so bad. I didn't know very much about taking overdoses and I only had enough money for 13 Anadin tablets, but it still warranted an overnight stay.

A few months went by and I went to my doctor. I used to suffer from crippling agoraphobia and panic attacks. He prescribed this drug called Anafranil, and I realised that if I took enough I would get on a high. So I bought a book which told me what symptoms I should be showing if it needs a bigger dose, and I started increasing the dose. The doctor was a fool because I'd go back like a month before the next prescription and ask for more. Then one time when I was drinking and I was on these tablets I had a major panic attack, and I was taken to hospital because I was getting twitches – tetany it's called. I pleaded with the nurses to take my tablets away and they just says, 'She's drunk that's all, she don't mean it'. So they didn't take them off me even though I was screaming for help. It got to the point where I was taking a tablet before every lesson at school otherwise I couldn't face the lesson. I was on an absolutely huge dose. I don't know what happened, but one day I just said 'Sod it', and I took the lot, about eight grams – 8000 milligrams of this drug – which was twice the fatal dose. This was in the middle of the afternoon, and in the evening my boyfriend came to take me out with his friends, but he said that I looked so tired he drove me straight home, and I cannot remember anything from taking the overdose until most of the way into my hospital stay.

When my boyfriend brought me back home I had a go at my mum and brother, apparently. I was screaming, swearing and shouting at them, telling them what I really thought of them. Then I went up to bed. Apparently the next morning I came down the stairs and said, 'Mum, I've got a migraine', and apparently I was so white she believed me and she sent me back up to bed. Then I started hallucinating that I couldn't move. I managed to get to the top of the stairs and I shouted down, 'Mum, Mum, I've taken all these tablets', and she says, 'Well just bloody well go and walk to the hospital'. This was my hallucination. But then I woke up and I was lying on the bed and I was paralysed. I could move my hands and my head but nothing else. And I went, 'Muuuum', and she came up. She said 'What? What do you want?' I said, 'Mum, it's the tablets'. She goes, 'What tablets? What are you talking about?' I said, 'I don't want to die Mum', which I did, but I said it because that was the only way to tell her what I'd done. The doctors came around and they shoved me straight into hospital. I was on a heart monitor. I know it's damaged my heart: my heart rate was approximately 130 beats a minute for a few weeks. It completely tired me out.

I was lying there having my ECG and I heard the nurses talking over me. One was saying 'What did she take?' and the other says I'd took tricyclics. She goes 'How many?' 'Oh, eight grams.' 'How long ago?' 'Nearly two days ago.' And she's going, 'Oh my God, she hasn't got much chance has she? All you've gotta do is hope. All we can do is try and stabilise her'. I was all right in the end. I was in for about five or six days, and my mother came to collect me. I had to be picked up because I was so young. She walked me through the hospital gates and she hit me, very very hard, so I fell on the floor, and she said, 'Don't you *ever* embarrass me like that again'. That's my mother, basically, that's what she's like. Things got worse after that, they really did, between me and her.

★ ★ ★

I went back to school, and then I resigned from the sixth form. It was one of the hardest decisions I've ever had to make. I had a career mapped out for me, but couldn't cope with the work and the stress. I went to work at McDonald's for a little while and then from McDonald's I went into being a waitress, which I stuck for about another eight months. Then I got a job interview with British Rail to work in the freight department. I beat about 2000 people for that job, but I blagged it didn't I? I got sacked after two months 'cos I was crap. I was 18, full of myself. Mum wasn't very happy because I wasn't paying her board and lodging, but the amount of money I was earning, she had all of it if she was going to do that, so I started not giving her money. I started going out at all hours of the day and night, started sleeping around. All I wanted was care really, but I did some very risky things. Just before my 18th birthday my mother chucked me out. I lived in pokey little bedsits for ages, but that's just by the by. I ain't seen my mother since I left.

I had three months when I was unemployed because I was waiting for an ET place to come up, then I went and worked in insurance. I left after the ET because they only offered me £5200 a year for running an insurance office, so I told them where to stick it. I got another insurance job, but that only lasted one day and two hours. The second day I was there I had a migraine and I had to go home, somebody drove me. I was thinking, 'I don't like these migraines, they're ruining my life, I can't go to work, I can't do anything'. When I got home the migraine vanished altogether, it was very strange the way it did that. But I already had it in my head what I wanted to do.

I'd already taken a few overdoses during that time, but nothing much. I took a bus up to the seaside near Morecambe Bay. There's a cliff there, and I went up onto this hillside by some trees, and I settled myself down and wrote a letter. That trip to Morecambe Bay was the most beautiful trip I ever had. Everything was sunshining and there was rabbits and birds and stuff. It was very strange, but I was so determined about what I wanted to do. I took an overdose of cold capsules because I'd got in my drug book that there was a dangerous ingredient in them. I took 80 of those and 10 temazepam, and I drank two and a half bottles of spirits. I don't know how I managed to drink that much, but that's what the police told me.

The next morning apparently I went to this woman's house and told her that I'd been attacked and that there was a man who'd been following me, whether that was hallucinated or real, I'm not sure. Anyway, I was in the police station, and somebody thought to ask me what on earth I was doing at 7 o'clock on a morning outside, asleep. I said, 'Oh I took an overdose'. So I was rushed to hospital and I suffered the most frightening time of my entire life. The first day I can't remember, apparently I was being sick. The second day I started to have very major hallucinations.

★ ★ ★

I hallucinated that there were people at the window on the third floor – identical boys doing an acrobatic pyramid outside my window. That wasn't too scary, but even when I closed the curtains I could still see the shadows – it was really weird. And then I had these jelly fish – big opaque jelly fish – all over the walls, all over the floor, all over the bed, everywhere. This is what I saw, and Oh bloody hell it was *awful*. I tried running from them and the nurses were dragging me back and putting me into bed because I was too weak to get up. And now there was water as well, lots of water everywhere. Have you ever seen that film, *The Abyss*? They've got an edge of water without anything supporting it, and that's what I saw. I saw the hospital being flooded, splashing and everything. Then the worst of it was the blisters and spiders. I formed blisters all over my body, huge ones. These blisters came up and they'd grow to a quite massive size, then they'd pop and hundreds of little red spiders'd go under my skin. I worked out what you had to do was hit the blisters before they popped then the spiders wouldn't come. So I was like this [*slapping herself*] all over my body, and my boyfriend came to see me and I was saying, 'Look! You can see 'em!'. He goes 'I can't see anything Steph, I'm sorry'. I'm going like this [*slaps her arm*], 'Look, you can even see a red mark where the blister was!' I've never been so terrified in my entire life. I didn't know that I was hallucinating at the time, it was reality. I had no insight at that point at all.

That carried on for a day. The next day they said, 'Look we're gonna send you to a place where they might be able to help you more'. Now I didn't know that meant a psychiatric hospital. The ambulance came to take me to

Morecambe. I had my nightie and dressing gown on and I was in a wheelchair. They took me into the day room of this hospital and I worked out what was going on. Of course everybody was staring at me and it freaked me out because I thought, 'Oh God, they're all loonies'. I didn't think about it at the time, but I thought later, 'If somebody came in in a wheelchair in a nightie and dressing gown in the middle of the day, would you look? Yes of course you would, you'd be interested to see what was going on'. But I took it to mean that all these people had terrible mental illnesses and they were going to start throwing things at me or talking to themselves. None of that happened, but I wasn't happy. I ran away from the ward twice and got picked up by the police. Eventually they discharged me after 10 days saying 'We cannot treat her at all'. So I went back to Preston on the Monday and my fiancé locked me in my bedsit and took away all the knives, all the things I could harm myself with. I got admitted to Preston General on the Friday and that was when I started talking. I was talking about the view of reality that I'd made for myself. I felt that aliens were controlling me; I thought they'd made me immortal; it's all in my mind – life is a hallucination basically – whatever you say or do doesn't really hurt anybody because it's not real. I started talking like that and the next thing I knew I was on Stelazine.

★ ★ ★

Altogether I was there for five months. They started putting me on more and more drugs because the first ones weren't working. But my life didn't get any better and I suffered some very bad mental abuse from some members of staff. They accused me of lying about my other reality. They said I was just saying it because I wanted to get mixed up in the services and I wanted to be looked after. Well I'd been conditioned as a child, if somebody accuses you of something and they're not going to believe you if you say not, you just say, 'Yes I did do it', to stop it. So I said 'Yes', and that is where it really started going bad – they disowned me. After few weeks I left the building and I took an overdose of aspirin.

About six hours later I went to the Samaritans. I was scared of dying, I didn't want it to hurt. So they took me to casualty and casualty says to me, 'Right, you can have a stomach wash-out or you can have ipecac' – now I'd never had either. I'd probably taken about five or six overdoses by then, but they didn't catch me in time to do a stomach pump. I said to the Samaritans 'Which one's better?' and they said 'Well apparently having your stomach washed out is a lot better', so I agreed. They did a stomach wash-out, which was the most horrendous experience of my life. I knew I'd damaged myself because the people who were doing it were saying, 'Oh look there's plenty of the red stuff here'. I'd started haemorrhaging because the aspirin takes away the coating of your stomach and makes it ulcerated.

I was sick during the stomach pump a couple of times, which was pretty horrendous. You've got quite a big tube down your neck and into your stomach and you're supposed to be able to breathe at the same time, but you cannot swallow and breathe at the same time can yer? So you've gotta try and breathe through your nose. They make you lie down, holding on to the bars of the trolley because you automatically try and pull the tube out because it's gagging you. They put it in and they say swallow, swallow, swallow. You swallow the tube, then you start gagging, and then you start being sick around the tube. Then there's the suction and there's pints and pints of water being put into your stomach and drained out, put in and drained out.

The two Samaritan ladies were great, they were waiting for me. After the stomach pump I felt fine, so I sent the Samaritans home, but then I started to be sick, major league sick. I was sick, sick and sick for days, that was what the aspirin had done to my stomach, and I kept having to drink this charcoal, which binds in your stomach, to help eliminate some of the drugs. So I was very, very sick for a long time and I was on a saline drip.

★ ★ ★

I stayed in medical for three days. I wasn't quite fit enough, but they transferred me back to psychiatric. They didn't really do anything, just said I was silly. Then about a week later they took me off all my medication, and a week after that I went out and overdosed on aspirin again. I was supposed to be on Zantac tablets to mend my stomach, and I had this antacid stuff, Gaviscon. I knew that if I overdosed on aspirin again, the aspirin would go straight through my system because I'd got no stomach, and that's what I wanted to do. I went out the hospital again, overdosed, and was caught. My favourite nurse on the ward was off duty and she found me under a subway popping aspirin in my mouth. She said she wanted me to go into hospital and I couldn't say no. Imagine what it would have been like for her, seeing me taking aspirin and then dying because I didn't go to hospital. I couldn't do that to a person. It's not what they thought in hospital, they thought I was a manipulator.

They got me into the casualty waiting room and they're saying, 'You're going to have a stomach pump', and I'm going, 'No way am I having a stomach pump, no siree. I'm leaving'. And I tried to go but this RMN stopped the door. She says, 'Right you've left me no choice, I'll have to detain you under section 5, sub-section 54' [of the Mental Health Act], which meant that she could stop me going anywhere for six hours or until the doctor came. Then the doctor came and put me on a section 5.2, which is 72 hours. So I smacked the nurse and I also smacked the registrar, and then the consultant came and I smacked the consultant. In the end I said I'd take ipecac. I was on the general ward for three days on a drip again, being given ipecac and charcoal and still being sick a lot.

I came off the medical ward and I went back to Winnick, the psychiatric ward. My GP came in as I was sat in the dayroom. He tapped me on the back and said, 'We'll get you sorted, don't worry'. Then this approved social worker came and I spoke to her for an hour. I was very suicidal, and I was very logical about why I was suicidal, and she says, 'Look I'm very sorry but I'm going to have to recommend that you're detained under a section 3'. Of course I was shattered. It was four days before my twentieth birthday, and a section 3 can wreck the rest of your life. You cannot do certain jobs, you cannot emigrate to certain countries if you've been on a section 3. I always wanted to emigrate to America, but now I will never be allowed to emigrate. I was put on this section 3 and that's when I started rebelling. I used to run away, take overdoses. I used to fight with the staff. I'd be trying to leave the hospital and they'd try and stop me leaving by physical means and I'd struggle, like most people would. I ended up in seclusion a few times to cool down.

What's seclusion like? I'll tell you what it's like. You get this small room, probably about the size of this room here, and on the floor is a mattress with special non-tearing sheets so you can't hang yourself. That's all you've got. You've got a window, but you cannot see out of it because its opaqued, there's a big plastic sheet on top of it. There's a plastic sheet in front of the mirror, and there's a door with a little spy hole. They open it, look in and then close it again. I was in there for about eight hours sometimes. That's when I managed to use my other personalities – what I used to call trancing out – so I don't remember those times.

It got to the point where if I wasn't in seclusion I'd be confined to my bed, and if I wasn't confined to my bed I'd be on special observation, which meant having a nurse with me 24 hours of every day. I began to rebel more and more because I was being controlled. Sometimes I used to abscond from the ward and I'd be brought back by the police. I went to Morecambe twice. The second time I ended up in a police cell, because I'd been staying at a bed and breakfast and I was getting a bit cross because I hadn't been brought back. So I rang up the police and dubbed myself. I said, 'Oh, I had this young girl around at our Guest House last night and she looked ever so depressed. She didn't have any bags with her or anything – I'm quite worried about her. She said she was going to have a walk down the seafront, maybe you can catch up with her there'. So the police came and I put up a fight, because that's what I wanted to do – I wanted to kick off – that's basically having a one-person riot. The policeman tried dragging me into the back of the van and there was me kicking and screaming, 'Get off you bastard'. It happened on a Saturday morning in Morecambe, there was tons of people there. It was quite a nice little sideshow for them really.

They took me back to the nick and made me stay in a police cell. I was going, 'I don't have to be in a police cell, I'm not a criminal, I'm here because I've got problems'. And they were going, 'No you're staying in the cells'. So every five minutes I go, 'I want to go to the toilet', so they let me out to go to the toilet, and then I go, 'I'm not going back in now'. They'd shove me in again and I'd go for it again. They eventually let me out when the staff from the hospital came to pick me up. I was saying, 'Why didn't I get a meal?' and they said, 'You refused it'. I said, 'I didn't refuse a meal'. They said, 'Yes you did. If we'd given it to you you'd only have thrown it around the room'. I said 'Bastard, I didn't refuse it'. He said, 'Your word against mine: you're the crazy one, I'm the policeman, who are they gonna believe?'

I'd been sick in the police station and I asked to see a doctor, but they said no. On the bus home I started to feel sick again, and I was sick into a little brown paper bag. One of them tried to throw it out of the window, but the wind caught it and splattered it onto the windscreen of the car coming up behind, and we were all laughing our heads off. By the time I got home I was depressed, and even though I'd been sick on the journey I didn't eat or drink for three days. By the third day I was so ill I couldn't get off the bed. My boyfriend came to see me and he went on at the staff, 'Has she got flu or something? She looks fucking awful. She needs urgent medical help'. The staff just told him to keep out of it. At the end of the third day my body took over against my will, went towards a cold tap and stuck my mouth underneath it, almost a reflex action. And of course then the staff thought they'd won didn't they? There's stupid little mind games going on in these places sometimes.

★ ★ ★

I spent five months there, two informal and three under the section 3. By that point they'd taken my money away, taken my shoes away; they took my clothes so that I wouldn't run away, and if I wanted to make a telephone call a member of the staff had to put the 10p in the thing. I was getting Giro checks and going out and cashing them and running away, so they stopped that as well. It used to become a game: Can I get away from them? I was double specialed sometimes [allocated two members of staff on observation]. Towards the end of my stay, my psychiatrist calls me in and says, 'Right, Steph. I don't think you ought to be in this hospital, but I cannot take you off your section because if you go and hurt yourself or commit suicide it's going to come back on me. So I suggest you go for a manager's review'.

This manager's tribunal came up. I got legal aid, so I had a top shot solicitor who specialised in mental health sections, and I had a mental health advocate, a volunteer. I told the advocate what I wanted to say. I said I wanted to go home, because I did at that point. I was thinking I could go home and take an overdose because I was so depressed that nothing was ever going to help me. So we put our case. I managed to say some of it and he finished it off, then the lawyer turned it around and made it into official speak. They give you the result about 15 minutes later on a piece of paper. They said they couldn't discharge me, but they were going to give me a week's trial leave and if that went all right I should be discharged.

I burst into tears 'cos I was so happy. I went around telling everybody, 'I'm going home. I'm going home. I'm never coming back'. I had to be in custody with my auntie and uncle who rented the flat I was living in, because you have to be discharged into the care of somebody when you're released like that.

★ ★ ★

The night before I was due to go back to the hospital I thought, 'I can't go back to that place. I don't want to stay away from it either. I just want to die'. So I made sure that Top of the Pops number one was the last thing I ever heard, and I went out to this place outside Preston, where I used to live. There was a large road nearby, and I went out to a dark stretch of the road. I made sure there was no street lights, made sure it was fast traffic, and it was raining so people wouldn't be able to brake in time. I says to myself, 'Well I'm looking for a car where there's nothing travelling behind it, nothing travelling the other side, because I don't want anybody to get hurt except me'. Then this car came along and I stepped in front of it.

I'll never forget that moment. It's in my mind all the time. I could see the headlights coming for me and I thought, 'This is it. If I die, great. If I'm seriously injured then at least somebody'll look after me in hospital or something'. I smashed the bonnet in, I smashed the windscreen in with this arm and was bounced into the middle of the road. I was still conscious and in a lot of pain; my arm hurt, my leg hurt, my foot hurt – I was run over on my foot. I got out of the middle of the road, crawled to the edge of the road and lay in the gutter in pain and in shock. The car stopped about a hundred yards up the road. All I could think of when I was in the middle of the road was, 'I'm going to get run over, I'm going to get crippled'.

The ambulance was called. The worst thing was, I couldn't believe it, in the cars following this car there was number one, a casualty nurse, and number two, a surgeon. After I've had a road accident to try and kill myself! God, you cannot win, can yer? A nurse and a surgeon. They could do anything, they could amputate your legs if necessary. They took me to hospital and then a psychiatric nurse came to see me, and pushed and pushed and pushed me until I told him that I'd done it on purpose. So they made me go back to the psychiatric ward the next day, me arm's in a sling and me leg and me foot were all bandaged up. I hadn't broken anything, but I'd sprained myself. I'd got run over by a car and I came off better than the car did.

★ ★ ★

Of course the nurses thought I'd manipulated the situation. They said I'd waited for a slow car to come along, I waited for it being an elderly couple. How the hell am I supposed to know whether it was an elderly couple in the car or not? It was pitch black. All I could see was the headlights. They put me in a single room with a nurse at the door. They didn't allow any patients to speak to me, the staff held me in contempt, and I was not allowed to speak to anybody for a week, in solitary. Then they put me back on my bed space and I was still not allowed to talk to anybody for another week – two weeks without talking to anybody. Not once did anybody say, 'Why did you do it?' They just said, 'Manipulator'. That was dreadful. I tell you, I was nearly psychotic by the time I came out of there 'cos you start hearing things if you've got nobody to speak to you and you're a chatterbox like me.

★ ★ ★

Obviously I was back on my section. It was just before Christmas '92. Then my fiancé left me; we'd been together for two years – he said he couldn't cope. It was the only time that the staff on that ward were ever nice to me, because he went and told them before he told me, and the staff were all over me. 'Would you like to come through and have a cup of tea in your bed space, Steph?' Staff don't make you cups of tea, no bloody hell. I was made a cup of tea. They weren't happy with my fiancé because they realised that that was very cruel – it's the worst thing you can do to somebody. That's really what precipitated me running away to Newcastle.

I went to Newcastle 'cos I've got an auntie who lives up there. By this time I was becoming very mentally ill. I rebelled against all signs of female authority because of my mother. I didn't connect these things, it just felt like symptoms all the time but the causes I was blind to. I had this very strange idea that I wanted to kidnap a Samaritan and scare her by stealing from her or something. I wasn't thinking straight. I'm ashamed of it, I really am. I told my auntie that I was discharged from hospital and she put me up. We went out that night and I met a young bloke. He said he'd pick me up the next night and go out for a party, which was good, but when he came round to pick me up the next day the police came knocking on the door and I got arrested. They found a knife in my bag.

★ ★ ★

Because I knew that if I got arrested by the police things were never going to get better, I'd put a razor blade under each insole of my shoes. When they put me in the interview room they took my shoes away, took the laces out and gave me them back – they didn't know about the razor blades. So when they locked me in this room deciding what they were going to do with me, I got one of the razor blades from my shoes and I slashed my wrists. Then for some reason I thought that if I waved a razor blade around they'd let me go, so I tapped on the window, and I goes, 'Can you come here please?' to the policewoman. 'Please, I wanna talk to yer.' She wouldn't come on her own, she came with another police officer. She opened the door and I was holding this razor blade. I said, 'Let me out you bastards, I'll fucking kill you I will'. They managed to disarm me, but while they were doing it the policeman got a fright, 'Oh shit, she's cut her wrists'. So he's panicking his little head off in case they're gonna get Hep B or AIDS or sommat. Then they sat down and they says, 'Why did you do that? Where did you get that razor blade from?' I says, 'I got it from the insole of my shoe'. They said, 'We don't think so. We think you had it somewhere else'. I goes, 'Are you saying what I think you're saying?' She says, 'Yes, we believe that you placed a razor blade in your vagina'. I went 'Uh! You don't believe me? Do you want me to bloody well show yer?' So I got me shoe off me foot, lifted out the insole, got the razor blade out, and I was so wound up by this stupid bloody bitch of a policewoman I slashed out at her with it. I don't think I hurt her very badly; I think she caught it with her hands. All I know is they disarmed me, dragged me by my hair into a bigger cell and called an ambulance. They bandaged my wrists and then they took me to hospital under like an armed guard. They were still trying to get the doctor to do an internal examination – I couldn't believe it. In the end they were going to take me to the Morpeth Special Care Unit, which is like an intensive care ward for mental health, but they contacted Winnick and Winnick said, 'We want her back'. The police weren't very happy because the staff at the hospital wanted to come in the morning. They said, 'We're not putting her in a cell overnight, she's obviously not well. We cannot keep her in a police cell, especially if she's like this when she wants to hurt herself' – it was all very positive. They weren't wanting to get rid of me because I was bad or they couldn't be bothered – they were thinking about me and how I felt.

So the police got an ambulance and drove me back down to Preston themselves. They put a policewoman in the ambulance with me, the same policewoman who I'd attacked, and she sat herself opposite me for the four-hour drive. They had me in a paper suit, a funny paper suit with a zip up it, it looks like it's made of nothing more than kitchen roll, but you could fit about three pregnant women in it, there's so much space. I had a jumper over that to keep me warm on the journey and I had handcuffs on as well so I couldn't hurt anybody. It was weird, I felt like a real strange criminal. And this policewoman who I'd attacked was so nice; we were having this great conversation, we were. She was really sympathetic to me and she talked to me for nearly all the way home. I was lucky. I could have been sent to Rampton for about eight years for attacking a policewoman like that with a razor blade. They could have called it attempted murder.

We got back to Preston and they put me in seclusion for three days. I lost a bit of that time as well because apparently I was extremely verbally and physically abusive to the staff, which I don't remember. Then they transferred me to what they call a semi-secure unit, basically locked wards. It was the day before Christmas Eve and I'd asked to speak to the nurse for some Christmas leave. He said, 'I'll speak to you after meds', and he took me into this small room after medication and said, 'Right, you're going to The Ashworth. Your things are already packed and the car's waiting outside'. Shocked? Bloody hell, I'd been assessed by him two weeks before, but I thought I'd got off.

★ ★ ★

I was on the bad ward over Christmas and New Year, the very disturbed locked ward. They call it the forensic ward because there's people in there on criminal conviction sections – people who need assessment for mental illness problems while they are awaiting trial and things like that – though sometimes they'd take on what they call social cases, which included me. I'd only been sent to The Ashworth for 14 days, but they decided to keep me because they thought they could help me. After the 14 days they sent me up to a ward called Hoxton, which is a young offenders' ward.

★ ★ ★

Hoxton Ward was fantastic. I got counselling every single day. I had a proper care plan you see, and they'd realised that I needed intensive counselling. So if I wanted to I could talk to somebody anytime – day or night – that was the way it worked. I was supposed to have a care plan in Winnick, but it was a standing joke on the ward. It wasn't a care plan, it was a riot act, which included time out if I misbehaved – that meant slung in a seclusion room really, but you can't say that in a care plan.

It took me about three or four months to get over the trauma of being in Winnick and the mental, physical and emotional torture that went on there. But they put me on an antidepressant that worked, I had a psychologist, and with the help of a really nice key worker, Laurie, a lot of things changed for me. Me and him got on so well. He once got called into question because I was in a ward meeting and they says, 'How do you feel about Laurie?' I says, 'Well I see him as a friend first and a nurse second'. Bloody hell, that was the wrong thing for me to say. They called him in and gave him a real hard time for that, saying, 'It's not supposed to be like this', and he told them all to fuck off. Not as such, but in his actions he did.

The most helpful incident in my whole psychiatric career was when I went for my assessment for Hoxton. I went to see this nurse and it was Laurie that I met. He was supposed to be doing a half-hour assessment on me. I was still there four and a half hours later, so was he. That's nearly four hours of his free time that he sat there talking to me. That was the single most helpful incident in my whole time of being a mental health user.

Oh, I must go back to something really important. Just before I was in Hoxton, I'd cut my wrists, right? In Hoxton I realised that there were girls who cut themselves and I thought it was stupid. The next thing I know I found out how relaxing it was, and these are the scars I've got all the way up my arms, up to my shoulders [*pulling her sleeve up to show me*]. It's got to the point where I cannot have any treatment ever for the rest of my life. Skin grafts wouldn't be appropriate, dermabrasion, which is taking off the top layer of skin, is too expensive, so is laser treatment. I did it for a year and I'm scarred for life now. I haven't worn a T-shirt in public since, that's why I'm sat here in long sleeves. In the summer it gets terrible. That was something that happened when I was in Hoxton, and I was still doing it when I came out.

★   ★   ★

I was lucky in a way that things got better after being in Hoxton. It wasn't all roses in there, bloody hell. I was whacked, I got shouted at, I had things thrown at me by other residents. It was not a bed of roses – it was very hard work. I spent about eight months in there and I left in August 1993. I resettled in Blackpool so that I wouldn't get admitted to Winnick. I started living in a Mind hostel with three other women. Then there was a muck-up with the community care because if you've been under a section 3, you've got to have a 117, which is a care plan for three months after you leave hospital. Unfortunately, when my three months finished I had no other contact, so I was from the middle of November to Christmas Eve with absolutely nobody. I ended up back in The Ashworth then for a fortnight, took an overdose yet again and had hallucinations. Nearly every overdose I've taken I've got hallucinations.

Eventually I got a social services resource counsellor, Steph her name was, same name as me. I met her on Christmas Eve, same year as I came out of hospital. We did a lot of work, Steph and me, 'specially on the sexual abuse and stuff. As I say, I never knew that I was being abused until about a year ago. They say false memory syndrome, I say a load of shit basically – a lot of people don't remember they're abused. It's the only way that your mind can cope, to blank off into another reality.

When I came out of Hoxton I was looking at my past and thinking, 'What can I do?' I thought, 'I'll become a psychologist because psychologists can change things'. I was wrong, 'cos they can't. I've spoken to a lot of psychologists now and they agree that it's impossible to change the system from the inside. But that autumn I tried to do some college work and I couldn't manage it. I was still looking for something to do with my time when I met Garth, who lived in another Mind hostel, and we hit it off very well. We were engaged within three weeks of meeting – I proposed. Sometimes you've just got to go out and get what you want [*laughing*]. He introduced me to the Mental Health User Forum – he was administrator at the time – and it was the answer to all my problems. I could change things and I've been doing that for a year now. We're all mental health users or ex-users and we support each other.

★ ★ ★

Working for the Mental Health User Forum has saved me really. It's something important to do in my life, even if it's just to help people who were treated like me or are still being treated like I was. Among other things we've talked to people from the Ambulance Trust and said, 'Why do people in ambulances treat people who've overdosed like shit? It's not going to help to be called silly little girls, as has happened'. But it's funny when I go around visiting hospital wards and stuff – I feel real scared. You get this terrible feeling that you're going to walk in through the door and they're going to lock the door and say, 'Huh, got you, sucker'. It's something that I've learned to do by looking at it semi-professionally.

We don't campaign as such, we inform and educate. I went to some six or seven national conferences last year, had meetings every week with different people. And we have changed things. For instance the city psychiatric hospital was going to be closed down and all 96 beds put into the Royal Infirmary. They were gonna have the ward quite high up in the building, and they were gonna have it right next to a main road, and behind the hospital was a railway line with a bridge. Until some mental health users went through it and said 'What the hell are you doing? If you're going to have people in there who are suicidal are you actually going to show them a map of where to go?' It's also difficult to control. How do you keep your eyes on 96 people in one hospital? So what they did in the end was halve the number of beds for the Royal Infirmary. The other 50 something places are going in the community. There's going to be a ward in each locality, 8–10 bedded units for acute patients, only a lot better than the old hospital. All except two are being built from scratch, and there's a mental health user on every single reprovision group. I'm a user rep now and I go to these meetings. I say what the users want, and 99 per cent of the time things get changed.

We also do training. We go out to social services, and we train people from students to consultant psychiatrists on what it's like to be a mental health user. I've got two training sessions this month, one of them to talk about my view of being on a section, and another to talk about my experiences of mental health generally. That's the same as I'm talking to you really, which is why I'm doing so well. The only other thing that I'd say is that at the beginning of my personal experience talks I do the shock bit. The shock bit is that I've over-dosed 25 times; I've had about 60, 70 stitches in my arms; I've been on 12 different psychiatric drugs. I've had Zimovane and Temazapan, which are both sleeping tablets; I've had propranalol, which can calm you down; I've had clomipramine, lofepramine, fluoxetine, Trazodone, those are all antide-pressants. I've been on Stelazine, I've been on Largactil, I've been on haloperidol, and I've been on procyclidine which is for side-effects.

The Melleril's all I am on at the moment, not even any sleeping tablets, because these tablets make me tired and they keep me stable as well. Now I'm against medication as a rule, but this one's made me feel better and that's been important to me. It's given me my life back. I feel like I didn't have a life some-times when I was a psychiatric patient, I felt like I was a number. P82275 I think my last number was – I know it as well as my Social Security number – it's dehumanising, really. You don't go into an orthopaedic ward and go, 'Oh look, this is Mr Green, he's a broken leg he is', but they do say, 'Here's Mr Green, he's a schizophrenic'. A person *isn't* an illness, a person *suffers* from an illness. The way they say schizophrenic, it's like once a schizophrenic always a schizophrenic. The diagnosis becomes the person.

Have I had a diagnosis? Oh, I've had practically all of them. I had schizo-phrenia at one point and I've had different personality disorders and anxiety neuroses, and post-traumatic stress disorder, depression. Before this lot of symptoms my full title was hysterical-personality-disorder-oblique-depres-sive-type illness. I cannot see myself without my medication in the near future. Maybe I will some day.

6.

I'd always thought crying was a sin: Diane Johnson

Slim and delicate, with cropped greying hair and a nervous manner, Diane reminds me of a bird. She'd be the sort of person who chain smoked, but she doesn't smoke. In fact, the house is squeaky clean and tidy. Diane is in her late 40s; she's held down a demanding job in marketing for 15 years, and today is a day off. Neatly turned out in a black skirt and cream sweater, she sits with her hands folded and her head on one side. Her looks belie a disturbing history, involving psychological and sexual abuse from a young age, from which she's now emerging with considerable determination. She begins by telling me about a bereavement workshop she recently attended.

Have you heard of Elizabeth Kubler Ross's work? You have, right, I don't need to describe it for you. If I'd known what it was going to be I probably wouldn't have gone. There's about 90, 100 people, they have about six, eight facilitators and all the work is done in front of everybody. When it started I thought, 'There's all these facilitators, all these people, so it must be that we split into little groups', and when I realised that anything that was going on was dealt with in the room, I thought, 'No way'. But it was very, very powerful. I found that when I went into that room I started to cry, and it was as though I was attached to a tap – tears pouring out of my eyes. Obviously something in that room was having an effect, even though nothing had really happened other than people introducing themselves.

You had to say three things about yourself, I can't remember exactly what they were, something you didn't like, something you did like. I said the thing I didn't like about myself was I wanted to die; I can't remember what my positive things were. Then they had mattress work, which is that people express how they feel on a mattress. What you gain from the workshop is that you're listening to other people having the courage to say why they're there, and people go there from the medical profession, people who've had bereavements, lost children, people with AIDS, and doctors who are at their wits' end, burnt out. So it's a really big mixture of people.

It was a very big turning point for me, because until then I'd always thought crying was a sin. Intellectually I knew it wasn't, but if I did cry I felt terrible about it. One thing they made very clear there was that there were no band-aids being given out. If you saw somebody what they called 'in feeling' you left them, so it was the very first time in my life I'd actually been allowed to cry. Nobody came to stop me or make me feel better, which often amounts to the same thing. There they just let you cry – so whatever was there could come out.

What was interesting was that at the very first meeting they had nearly a hundred chairs in the room, and gradually they took the chairs out and there were fewer chairs and more cushions on the floor. It was a five-day workshop, and as the days wore on I gradually went nearer and nearer the front. I didn't get onto the mat until right near the very end, and when I did I couldn't do anything. I just sat there, and I said to this woman facilitator, 'I can't say anything, I feel dead'. She said to me, 'What do you want?' And it came out that I felt like screaming, but I couldn't scream, so she said to everybody in the room, 'Right, Diane wants to scream but she can't, so I want you to help her'. She got everybody in the room to scream so that I could scream, and once I started to open up I was amazed at what came out. I thought somewhere along the line I was going to get in touch with grieving about my father, because I'd never grieved about him, but something else came out, and that was the fact that I'd been sexually abused as a child, and sexually abused as an adult by a therapist I'd gone to see.

★ ★ ★

I had such a bad time when I was a child. My father never sexually abused me, but he used to beat me up. He was shell shocked from World War II and he'd been in hospital for many years. My brother was born when I was two-and-a-half and then a year later they had my sister, and I suppose my father couldn't cope, so I used to get farmed out. I got sent to my great uncle, my mother's uncle; he had a wife who was very neurotic and they had no children, and he used to come into my bedroom at night. He used to buy me things during the day, which was very confusing: I was a little girl during the day and not a little girl at night. So I was very sexually experienced as a young child. The other person was a young man who worked for my father. My father had a furniture shop, and I don't know how it started with this guy, all I know is that we used to have sex. I was about five and he must have been 15, 16. I remember going upstairs to the storeroom, I remember him lying on top of me, and I remember him going inside, so it was definitely intercourse with him, and somewhere along the line I knew it was wrong. I don't know how I knew, but I remember one day he was calling me up to where he was and I wouldn't go, so I stopped that.

I think what was happening to me made me quite a tearful child, but my parents were quite superficial and they couldn't cope with emotion at all. 'God will punish you', they used to say, 'God will punish you'. Then my mother gave birth to another child when I was 11 and I was incredibly jealous of this child – though I loved her as well. She died when she was five weeks old. I remember my parents saying to me, 'God punished us because you used to cry so much'. At that age you take things like that on board, and it was like having a knife stuck inside me. I suppose how I look on it is that from age 0 to 10 my life was just a nightmare. I never had any childhood at all.

I left home when I was 17 and went to live in Canada. This was 1963; thirty years ago. My friends were gobsmacked because I was very quiet and shy, and it was very unusual then for a parent to let a child go away for years. But I was pushed out of the house, I call it oiled out, I wasn't actually forced out with a shotgun but they wanted me out. I married a Canadian guy I met coming back from Canada when I was 20. I had a sixth sense that he wasn't right, but my parents were adamant that I get married to him. I didn't know anything about him or his family, and my parents didn't check into it. He was actually addicted to gambling.

★ ★ ★

My husband was very emotionally abusive. We lived in Canada and I didn't know anybody. He wasn't a social person, so at the beginning it was very much him and me, and that was okay with me because I had his undivided attention, which was something I'd never had from anybody. But he gradually took me over. I ate what he said, dressed in what he said, it even got to the stage of him telling me when I could change my sanitary towels – he went into the loo one day and discovered there wasn't enough blood on one of them. He was a real miser. When he was courting me I remember he bought me an *enormous* bottle of Rive Gauche, the biggest one he could buy. At first I thought, 'That's really nice', but later I realised it was because it was more economical to buy a big bottle than a little one – that was his mentality.

I was four years in Canada that time, and the marriage wasn't consummated for three years. My husband said it was my fault and I believed him. He said I was neurotic and he would just masturbate on me and that was accepted. But I knew it wasn't right and I felt terrible about myself – I thought I was a freak of nature, I thought I had no opening. When I'd been married for nearly a year I phoned up the family planning clinic – I didn't know what else to do. I was blabbering on on the phone, and then at the end I said my marriage hadn't been consummated, so they suggested I went to special counselling. Well that was a terrible thing. I went to this agency, managed to tell them what was wrong; they sent me to a doctor and the doctor tried to examine me and it was just awful. I remember the doctor going like that to me [clenching fist]. He said, 'That's what you're doing. It's because you're in a new country, a new job, a new marriage. Go away and relax'. So I went away thinking, 'Well it *is* all my fault'.

What saved my life was an article in the newspaper. It was about testing and advisement centres all over Canada, and they rated Toronto University very highly. Well I thought it would be brilliant for my husband, because he'd been in the armed forces, and when he came out, to cut a long story short, he became a plumber, but he'd left that job and he was floating around, he didn't have proper employment. So I thought if he was doing a job that he really liked maybe it would help our marriage. But in the end the both of us did it together, and what came out was that they rated me in the top percentage of my age group, the top six per cent of intelligence. Well I was gobsmacked because I'd left school when I was 15, I never passed the 11-plus, so I didn't rate myself in any way, shape or form. They said that I had problems that were holding me back, and if I wanted to sort them out they would help me.

Well my test was much better than my husband's and he didn't like that. But what also came out was that I suddenly became aware that my husband didn't think anything was wrong. Yet there *was* something wrong, even if it was all my fault. So I went to the agency that the University had recommended, and it was brilliant. Right at the very end I spoke to the woman there about the non-consummation of the marriage, and she said, 'When you first came and we were talking I wondered why you were here, because there's nothing wrong with you'. (I'm very good. I've learned over the years to keep everything inside, so I'll present one face to the public and I'll be dying inside.) She said, 'What we'd like you to do is go to a gynaecologist'.

I went to see this gynaecologist on a Saturday, on my own, and his wife was there. She was a social worker or something, they had trained with Masters and Johnson, and there was just the three of us in the office. He said, 'I don't care how long it takes, you are going to examine yourself, because otherwise you are not going to believe me'. So he had these instruments: a very small instrument, then a bigger one and a bigger one, and it took hours. His wife held my hand while I put these instruments inside me, and eventually I put the big one in; I was crying my eyes out because I'd thought I had no opening. Afterwards I was meeting my husband in town. I had a woollen dress on with a belt and I bloused it over. He said to me, 'Pull your dress down, don't blouse it over'. Well in the past I would have pulled it down, and I said, 'No I won't'. I can't remember what happened after that, whether he walked away from me in a temper or what, but that was the beginning of the end of my marriage.

★ ★ ★

After I realised I had an opening we were able to have sex. But it was awful, it was like nothing. It reminded me of being a child, just lying there and no feeling, no passion. By then I knew we needed help, and my husband agreed to come and see this one particular therapist, this man who used to write a magazine advice column. So before the marriage ended we went for this sort of marriage guidance, and gradually I realised that that was it. It was really weird because whereas I'd always thought that I was the weak one and he was the strong one, it ended up that he was the weak one. After I left him he went through various phases: he'd crawl to me on his hands and knees and say he'd do anything if I would come back. Then he'd feign illness, he was dying, he had cancer or a heart condition. And he used to send the most weird letters to me at work, long letters, because after I left him he never knew where I lived. He didn't write on paper, he'd write on flyers like you get through the letter box, in between the lines and down the sides. It took me a long time to get away from him. In the end I managed to get him to sign a form that would entitle me to get a Mexican divorce, and I flew to Mexico.

After the divorce I got engaged to somebody who was totally the opposite of my husband. He was overweight whereas my husband exercised and was a perfectionist. But what was really awful about the engagement was that I was introduced to this man by my therapist – it was one of his patients and he set it all up. I was manipulated right along the way. When I first went out with Ian I was frigid. Well, I'd been frigid as far as my husband was concerned, so I just assumed I was frigid and there was no physical contact. Then he held my hand one day, after I'd been going out with him for quite a while, and it was as though an electric shock went through me. That night he kissed me for the first time, and suddenly I didn't know what was happening to me – and he got a shock as well. Later on I found out that he was telling the doctor about what was happening with us sexually, and I felt very betrayed. I thought it was voyeurism. There were lots of other things that were just not nice and that to this day I don't really understand. All I know is that I was very lucky to get out.

I didn't really want to be engaged, because much as I liked being with Ian I wasn't ready. The engagement ring was a surprise. He said he wanted to marry me and I said, 'No', and then he turned up with an engagement ring. I felt that if I didn't say, 'Yes', I would lose him. But I went from one manipulative relationship into another. He gradually wanted me to dress in a certain way, do certain things. I wouldn't set a date for the wedding. And his family, who had accepted me at first, got very angry at me. Then he put a deposit on a house without me being there and I was angry at him – I thought it was terrible. So we had this disagreement, and that was the last time I ever saw him. I'd gone to therapy, he was supposed to pick me up, and he didn't turn up. I was waiting on the pavement for a long time. I found out later that the doctor knew he wasn't going to come, but he didn't tell me. Then I received a letter from him saying that he couldn't cope and he just had to get away, and I was demented. I wrote a letter saying I was sorry, I'd do anything. I tried to phone to find out where he was, and nobody would tell me. And I became ill in a strange way: I had a lump in my throat and nothing would go past it.

I carried on seeing this therapist, and that was when he started to take advantage of me. That was just a total nightmare, because I reacted in the same way as I had when I was a child – just kept very still and pretended it wasn't happening. As far as I remember there was no sex with this man, he just touched me and made me touch him. But it was awful, so when I came back to England again in my late 20s, I was ill.

★ ★ ★

Then I had a nervous breakdown. It started a year or so after my mother died: I was itchy all over my body and the doctor gave me some pills which I didn't like taking. Eventually I was referred to the psychiatric hospital; I had problems with checking, I couldn't stop checking things, everything had to be in a certain place, it was just a nightmare. I saw a psychologist for about two years and he gave me various exercises when he'd come to my home and mess things up and I had to leave them, but I think he eventually realised it was more than that. Then he moved on and I saw a hospital psychiatrist as an outpatient and had drugs. I hated taking the drugs. I was drugged for years, and my mouth was always dry. Then I got really bad a few years later and I was admitted for about a month. I was admitted twice over a period of three years, and after that first time I saw a psychiatrist once a week for a while. Then I had to go to hospital to have a minor operation and I started to go really downhill.

★ ★ ★

The second time I was in I had ECT, quite a lot of courses of ECT. I don't think it helped, and it also affects your memory, but who knows? When I was really bad my sister phoned around, and she spoke to a friend of the family who's a psychiatrist and he said, 'If it was me I'd have the ECT'. Maybe I would have been worse, maybe I would have been dead if I hadn't had it. If I knew then what I know now I wouldn't have had it, but I was a different person then.

I was off work for six months. Then my psychiatrist left and a new one took over and this new doctor was very good for me, because until then I'd gone through a phase of phoning them all the time. I'd drive them mad, it was like an obsession – I had to hear their voice otherwise I'd feel as though I couldn't cope. This psychiatrist was very tough. He said to me, 'I know you need to phone us, that's fine, but we'll make a contract. If you phone me I will speak to you, but it will have to come out of the time I see you as I don't have that much time to spare'. So while in the past I knew they'd get irritated, but nobody would ever say anything, he brought it up front and it made sense to me – I felt as though I was being heard and seen. Of course I didn't like it – I felt humiliated – but I respected him for being honest with me. I told him I didn't like him, and he said that was fine but, he said, 'You don't know me'. So that was the beginning of the beginning for me. This psychiatrist told me later that when I'd first started seeing him I was a child, and gradually over the years I started to grow up.

★ ★ ★

I started to take more responsibility for myself in my 40s, by not just relying on the National Health Service to help me. I went to group therapy for quite a number of years, and I decided when I went into group therapy that I was going to do things for myself as well. So I started looking, and that's when I started to go on different workshops and read books and so on. I'd lost confidence in the written word, even talking – it was amazing how I held down a job all that time. I feel I've gained so much from listening to people on the radio and television and reading books. When I heard about this I thought, 'Well if I've got something to say, even if it helps one person, then how can I help?' So as much as I feel totally sick about doing this, I couldn't say no; there wouldn't be any hesitation.

I've found the workshops have been very helpful, and friends too. Realising for example, through the Elizabeth Kubler Ross workshop, that it's not a sin to have bad feelings, that it's best to accept them. One big thing I've learned is that you can actually feel good and bad at the same time. So whereas in the past I'd have been terrified of negative feelings and tried to push them away, now I try to make friends with my negative side and then I can function positively – I don't get paralysed. I allow myself to feel what I'm feeling. And that's where Cheryl is great, we've become close friends, and she's very accepting of me. We can talk about anything under the sun in depth or just skim the surface, and we're very honest – if I'm not in the mood or she's not in the mood, we'll be very upfront about how we feel.

I've got other friends too, besides Cheryl. In my 30s I only had friends from my childhood, but once I started to be OK some of them were very threatened and they didn't like it that I'd got a mind of my own. So in my 40s I started to make new friends. It started when my sister phoned up and said that there was an advert in the paper for a local singles group, why didn't I go along? That was my very first venture out on my own, socially, for about 10 years, and there was a girl there who I'm still friends with today. Then through her I met other people and I started to branch out. I do like people and I find I can have more invitations than I can cope with. I don't have enough time to do all the things I'd like to do. I'd say that until the turning point in starting the workshops it was as though my life was black and white, and now I've got colour.

The diary of Anne Frank was the first book that really helped me when I was a young girl. And then *Reader's Digest, Time* magazine, and the self-help books really: *The Road Less Travelled; Feel the Fear but Do it Anyway; Begin It Now. The Courage to Heal* – that's for women survivors of sexual abuse – I found very enlightening. I thought at the time that if I'd read that book years ago I wouldn't have suffered as much as I did, I wouldn't have felt so alone. I thought I was the only one who'd ever had sexual abuse as a child, and as far as the therapist was concerned I thought I was the only person in the whole wide world. When I found out that it happened to other women and it was very common it made me feel a bit more normal.

I'll tell you what did help at one workshop I went to. It was a creativity workshop and the workshop leader had me do an exercise. Everyone had to do a two-minute piece, and I chose to do a poem. Afterwards he said, 'Now are you willing to take a chance?' I said, 'Fine'. He got all the men in the room to form a semi-circle round me, and I had to say this poem and then he made them step closer and closer to me and suddenly, when they were very close, I became paralysed from my neck downwards, I *could not move* at all. He held my hand and talked me out of it and it was like a breakthrough really, something very profound happened to me after that. I think that's how I'd coped with being abused as a child: I'd lived in my head and my body didn't exist, and in that workshop it was as though my body and my head came together. That workshop helped to put me more in touch with my sexuality and be less frightened of it. I'm not there yet, but compared to the way I was years ago I'm very different. Especially when I started to wear different colours. There was a period of time when I couldn't wear anything but black, and when I started wearing vibrant colours it took some getting used to.

★ ★ ★

Time-wise my job is very demanding, very stressful, but I ride it. I've survived 11 years, though I've had a lot of problems. What was awful was that I was in my previous job for 10 years and I had a tough time there. Before I left that job I went for an interview with one of the major UK PR and marketing agencies and I was very upfront about having psychiatric treatment, I didn't hide it. I was offered the job and I was delighted. Then I did something very foolish: I gave in my notice before I'd had my letter of confirmation and I left. I gave myself a week's holiday, and during that week I got a phone call from the man at the agency who'd told me I'd got the job and he was pig sick. He said, 'I'm really sorry, the company's getting cold feet, they're worried about you and you'll have to come in and see the company doctor'. I thought, 'Oh my God'. I had no job, and how do I explain to any future employee why I left my other job? The whole thing was just a nightmare. I wrote a piece about it actually:

> It was a long and difficult interview. It didn't start off too well. I accidentally walked into the room before the doctor was ready for me and he impatiently looked up at the ceiling in exasperation. My stomach sank. I told myself once again that I had nothing to be ashamed of and tried to compose myself in readiness for the interview.
>
> I was taken aback by the doctor's extreme lack of sensitivity. He conducted the interview in such an aggressive manner that even the attending nurse seemed embarrassed. The doctor made it crystal clear that he was reluctant to recommend that the company employ me, as he was unsure of my ability to cope with the exacting demands of the job. This attitude only had the effect of making me more determined than ever to make a success of the interview and hopefully the job. Finally, he agreed to let me start work on a two-month trial period. Eventually, when I did go back, he was amazed that I had coped so well.

★ ★ ★

Well, I worked my socks off. I felt as though I owed it to everybody who had ever had any mental illness: if I didn't do well, they'd never employ anybody again. But that wasn't the end of my problems by any means. In the office where I worked there was a queen bee who disliked me, and she had her entourage. She made life a nightmare for me for years. There used to be problems with noise: I can't work with a lot of background noise and they liked to have the radio on. And they never included me in anything. My psychiatrist said to me once, 'It's a bit like a cold war – they know what's going on, you know what's going on, but nobody's saying anything'. What you can do is go to the weakest link and ask this person what's going on'. So I went to this one girl and asked her, 'Why aren't you friendly towards me? Why don't you want anything to do with me?' Well, she just screamed at me, 'I don't want to talk to you, I don't want to know you'. And I was hysterical; I went back to work crying. Quite a few times during the first few years I was called up to personnel: 'Why are you crying in the Department? You're depressing people', and 'Do you want to go home?' I always knew I didn't want to go home because I thought if I did it would be ammunition for them.

Then one day I went into work early in the morning, and I went up to the queen bee and said to her, 'Why are you not nice to me? For what reason?', and she got very angry with me and started pushing me down the corridor. It was like being hit – I don't know if you've ever been hit by anybody, but it's awful – it really distressed me. When I went back in the office one of the junior managers took me aside and said, 'What's wrong? Whatever you tell me is in confidence'. So I told her, but it wasn't in confidence and it went round the office that I was a snitch and then I was sent to Coventry – *nobody* would talk to me. And this went on for a few weeks until the management called her and me in for interview and they said to me that it could be a police matter because I was accusing her of assault. I said, 'I don't want the police involved, because I don't believe that she got out of bed in the morning to hit me, I think she did it on the spur of the moment and I'm prepared just to leave it be'. But they demoted me, put me on another section, and I was very upset about that. Then this girl left. Her friend was promoted to the manager position and she wanted me out and made no bones about it.

But then most amazing thing happened in the office. Gradually once this queen bee left the others began to see me in a different light, and they started to complain about how I was being treated. By then I'd reached the end of my tether, and I remember one Friday I came home from work and I was crying all night. I phoned the Samaritans, I couldn't stop crying. I was still crying the next day, I just felt I was dying: it was the sheer accumulation of it; it had gone on for years. I thought, 'I can't go back there anymore', and I phoned my doctor on the Saturday and went to see her. I thought she'd send me back to hospital or put me on tranquillisers, but she didn't. She said to me, 'You wouldn't be working in that job for that many years if you didn't know what you were doing. You can do that job – and you can go into work on Monday'. Well, I went into work on the Monday and they changed. I don't know whether she phoned them or what happened, but that manager left me alone.

★ ★ ★

What I learned from that experience is how important it is to be upfront with your emotions and upfront about what's going on – don't let cold wars start. Now in my job I'm very protective of new people who come in. I'd never let what happened to me happen to anybody else. So if anybody new comes into the department…and going into marketing can be very intimidating, especially here, because it's a big office, each one is a personality plus and they're very intolerant…if anybody new comes in, and anybody says, 'Oh God look at her', I say, 'Look she's new, so what if she's talking too loud or whatever. You don't know what's going through her mind, maybe she's not sure how to act'. And I make it very clear, if it's humour below the belt I won't let them get away with it. I'll nip it right in the bud, even to the extent that I'll actually say to them, 'If you carry on with this I'm going to report you'.

I like working in marketing. I like the people I work with, they're very upfront and very zany. I like talking to people, and I like the creativity that's involved. I'm actually an enigma here because I'm in my 40s and I got my job without having a university degree, I got it on the strength of my personality or whatever. As far as education is concerned, maybe my life is more difficult financially and maybe I'd have got a lot of pleasure from learning, but there's also something to be said for learning things from where you are, not being *told* how to learn. I suppose at the end of the day I don't wish that anything that ever happened to me hadn't happened, because who I am today is everything that's ever happened to me. All I want to do now is go on from where I am, take advantage of what's available and do the best I can.

7.

Oops, there goes the telly: Lesley Tutt

The front door opens on to a reception area, and this is where we sit down to talk since it's the only part of the house where smoking is allowed. Lesley is plump, 30-something, friendly, smiling, and down-to-earth. I like her enormously straight away. She has her own flat now, but this is the family home where she grew up and her mum still lives. Relatives smile out of family photographs on the bookshelves and walls. In pride of place is a picture of Lesley at her graduation ceremony. It's been a tough journey for her. Lesley suffered abuse throughout her childhood, and developed many self-destructive behaviours that it's taken a great deal of hard work to combat.

I think my mental health problems became apparent when I was very young, around 11 or 12. I'd had a school change and left all my school friends behind, so that was very unsettling. But there was a lot of dynamics going on in the house as well, my father was an extremely difficult person to live with, a tyrannical person. He really dominated all of us in one form or another. He was very much a Jekyll and Hyde character, and you never knew when he was going to explode; he'd get into these explosive moods where he would scream and shout and really go puce. All in all it was an extremely difficult environment to live in.

I arrived at this big school knowing nobody at all. I can only remember being desperately unhappy and feeling that I didn't have any control over my life. In the home my dad's behaviour was all about control. Certainly he wasn't averse to hitting us – not just me but the lads as well. Then somewhere around about the age of 11, 12, I started to get a load of labels attached to me: 'attention seeker', 'disturbed', whatever. I was just a class clown; I would make people laugh all the time, so I suppose there was an element of attention seeking in it.

I was referred eventually to my GP who placed me on Valium. I continued to have panic attacks. Then the Valium at some point was replaced by amitriptyline, and not long after that by Ativan, lorazepam. So it was a very early process for me, being allocated tablets and medication to curb my behaviour. I didn't at that point understand what was going on. Just felt really, really depressed. When I was about 13 I tried to kill myself and I ended up in hospital. And when I was about 14 I started to cut myself with a razor blade. My behaviour became so alarming at one time that the teachers removed me from class. I was taken out of lessons for about 18 months and placed in a classroom on my own. I wasn't allowed to play with the other children; I wasn't allowed to go out during the break. I think it was about that time I really started labelling myself. I felt very much that everything was somehow my fault, and therefore I must be bad. Being in that classroom on my own I remember feeling intensely isolated and depressed. My mum was regularly getting called to the school, but within that 18 months she told me she wasn't aware that I was taken out of the lessons, and as soon as she found out she removed me from the school and refused to let me go back.

★ ★ ★

My first admission to a psychiatric ward was when I was 15. It was a local psychiatric unit at the general hospital. I remember that the psychiatrist there was very intolerant of me and saw me as an attention seeker and wasting her time. I was also referred at some point to an educational psychologist and a child psychiatrist, but I only have vague recollections of this. I remember feeling that this educational psychologist was particularly stupid because she kept asking me stupid questions and making me do silly little games.

I remember the day I went into psychiatric hospital. They had a sick bay at school and I couldn't stop crying. I think there was a build-up of me trying to act normal that maybe lasted for about six or seven months. I was trying to suppress a lot of very unhappy feelings so that I would be normal like everybody else, and that became so overwhelming for me at this point that I just broke down. I remember they called for my mum. My mum took me home, the GP was called and I was carted up to this psychiatric hospital where I stayed for about two or three weeks. I think I was just relieved that I was away from home. It was like a haven for me.

Home was scary all the time because you never knew when my dad was going to erupt, when he was just going to come in from work and start screaming. I could always cope with being hit periodically. It was the waiting to see whether you were going to get hit. My dad was very skilled at manipulating people's fear. He was a very oppressive man, on occasion very violent and certainly always verbally violent. I was always totally thick, I was stupid – gormless was a regular word I heard; it was just continuous. He was the same with my mum, what did she know? She knew nothing. My mum and I don't talk about this much nowadays, but when we do it's about how my dad really made us feel valueless. He was a very weird character – a street angel and a house devil. Everybody said what a lovely man he was and the life and soul of the party. I remember when I was being difficult at school my dad saying, 'You'll go to a home'. In a way that made my behaviour worse, because that was exactly what I wanted – to be removed from all this.

When I left school at 16 I didn't have any qualifications because I'd missed so much schoolwork. I was in hospital when they were taking the mocks, but I wouldn't have been educationally up to scratch anyway. I had a boyfriend then for about four years. We were more like friends as far as I was concerned. But I think Paul wanted a girlfriend, and in terms of sex I couldn't handle that at all, it really scared me, I didn't feel comfortable with the intimacy of a relationship, so there was very much a distance and we used to row about that all the time.

★ ★ ★

Straight from school I went to commercial college and learned to type, then I worked for a bank for a couple of years. There was still this misery which bubbled away underneath no matter what I was doing. I was fine if I was active and absorbed in other things or other people, but five minutes on my own and there was this discomfort with myself.

Eventually I left the bank and left Merseyside and went to Wales to work with people with learning disabilities. I'd never ever come across anybody with any kind of disability and it was a live-in job. I left mostly to get away from home and partly because I'd become increasingly unhappy with the demands for intimacy, which I couldn't cope with. Paul had become quite abusive, he'd started drinking quite heavily and on one occasion hit as well, so I wanted to get away from that. And actually it was quite a nice period in my life because I was so involved in these people and I really liked my work, I was quite happy there. I liked the commune atmosphere, where everyone mucked in. For me it was like a family, we were very supportive of each other. But they had a fire there and the building was completely gutted, so I lost my job.

I came back and worked in the Civil Service for about two years, typing in the Official Receiver's office. It was really boring and made me very depressed because there were mass redundancies – we were just hitting the recession. And I was living at home. I think after two years it was just intolerable. So eventually I left to work in Switzerland. I'd been on a trip there the year before, and I thought I'd like to go for a job. So I went to night school and learned a working knowledge of German and wrote to this lady I'd spoken to in a hotel there, 'Please can I come and work?' and she said, 'Yes', and sent me a contract and I went.

I thought I would be happy if I went somewhere as far away from the family stress as possible, but it didn't quite work like that. I stayed in a beauti-ful place, a Swiss chalet in a little village about an hour away from Lucerne. When I first arrived there I thought, 'This is *so* peaceful, I can just feel it in my bones I'm going to be happy here'. Then after the novelty and the beauty of the place wore off I was ferribly unhappy because I felt so *intensely* isolated. I was *totally* exploited and worked ridiculously long hours for very little money, and I started what developed into a really bad drinking problem. I started to drink, not excessively, but consistently, and it was enough to set me off; that this was a comforting kind of thing and slightly took the edge off my misery. Then an English girl came to work in the hotel a couple of doors down. At last I had a friend.

★ ★ ★

I think it was at that time that I pressed my own self-destruct button. Certainly we'd drink, and although I was happy to see somebody who I had something in common with, in a way it was probably the worst thing that could have happened because we were drinking partners then. So from drinking privately on my own in small amounts, we would go out all the time and get really, really drunk. I'd finish my shift at 10 o'clock, and perhaps I'd been on from 7.30 and I was just exhausted. I'd be going off for Julie who finished much earlier than me, who was treated much better than me, and we'd go out and get drunk for the rest of the night.

One night we went to this club with some Yugoslavian people who spoke a little bit of English and a little bit of German, so between us we were able to communicate. I got drunker and drunker and Julie got drunker and drunker, and I don't remember much of what happened, but at one point in the evening I was raped – not by the people we were with, we got lost from them somewhere in the middle of nowhere. We were wandering around in the early hours trying to find a phone box so we could get a taxi to take us home, and we stopped and asked this policeman. I was quickly sobering up at this point, particularly as I felt responsible for Julie, who was a few years younger than me and was really scared. We followed the directions this policeman had given us and couldn't find the phone so we headed back, and just as we were coming to a corner this car stopped and one of the fellows in the car asked me if we needed any help. I said we were trying to find a phone. 'We'll give you a lift', he said. Then this policeman we'd just spoken to came up and obviously knew these people. He said, 'These lads will take you to the train station'. I remember particularly asking, 'Are we safe?' in German, and he said, 'You're fine'. I must say there is no way I would have gone in a car had I not felt that it was safe. The long and short of it was that this man apparently wasn't a policeman, he was a night watchman. He told the police he knew nothing about it and hadn't met us – he lied. But the end of the story was that I spent about four days in hospital, just totally destroyed.

★ ★ ★

I woke up in this ward in a lock-up hospital. Apparently Julie had told them that I'd been in hospital earlier in the year. (I think perhaps the reason they'd asked her was that I couldn't speak and they associated that with a breakdown. That's how I've made sense of it, with the bits and pieces of information I've got.) All I remember of the rape is feeling that this man was strangling me and that I was dying. Julie said that the other fellow hadn't hurt her – he'd got a bit scared and backed off. She said I was lying there and she was trying to wake me up and I just cried. She wandered off looking for somewhere to get help and eventually came across some houses. She'd knocked these people up and she didn't speak any German so she had to direct them to me. I remember the police coming and interviewing me. I also remember that they took me to another hospital for a gynaecological examination and I remember lying on this bed with my legs up in these stirrups and feeling totally exposed, really slimy, while this man poked about. It was absolutely horrible, probably worse than anything that's ever happened to me. I remember crying and crying and crying, 'I want my mum'.

My elder brother Alan and my mum came to bring me home. Apparently I'd been there about four days before they knew I was there. My dad picked us up at the airport and he hugged me but he wouldn't look at me, and it made me feel like it was my fault for causing more hassle. He wouldn't look at me for about five or six days.

Julie wrote to me afterwards and her letter was really distressing. She wrote that she'd stayed overnight in the hospital and the police had come and woken her up at 3 o'clock in the morning. They had a suspect and took her down to the police station to identify him, but she couldn't remember because (a) we'd both had a lot to drink and (b) it was very dark and very traumatic. But she said in her letter that she felt responsible, it was *so* sad. I wish I'd had time to see her later on, you know it wasn't her fault, it was no-one's fault at all really. I feel a bit sad now. Can we stop a minute?

★ ★ ★

I think I had a blank for a couple of years because I don't remember much. I remember this GP saying to me when I came back 'You know your mind is not a blackboard; you can't just erase the bad bits', and I felt a bit comforted by that. My periods stopped for about three months, and I remember him trying to reassure me about the periods; it may well be just a massive shock to my system. It was really odd because I wanted to stay at home for the first time in my life: it felt secure. My dad treated me differently as well – he was a lot more tolerant of me – but it all went completely over my head.

I got a job working in a hostel for people with learning disabilities again. It was only part-time, but I spent a lot of my own time. I really loved it. I bought myself a bike and cycled to work every day. Then I got a full-time job with the health authority in a group home and I was really happy there. I really liked the people I was working with and I liked my colleagues as well. It was part of the community care movement in the early days. These people had all come out from a big institution for mental and physical handicap with hospital haircuts and trousers up their legs somewhere, and we put so much work into getting them to look normal even, it was really nice in terms of seeing them develop. We had a lot of support between the three support workers, which was really good, and I was quite settled in that I was really absorbed in my work. With the exception of the last few years I think that was about as stable as I'd ever been.

Whatever spare time I had I went to night school. I'd applied for nurse training with mental handicap so I had to do what is called a GNC I think. I passed that at SEN level and went off to do my training at a hospital in Brighton. I got involved almost immediately with this male student nurse in our class and we rowed all the time. We really didn't like each other very much, but we seemed to cling together maybe because we were that little bit older than the rest of the school. We slept together and that was quite comforting because there was never any demand for sex. He was a really weird person actually: when we were on our own he was really tender and put no pressure on me to do anything that I didn't want to do, yet when he was around other people he would show off all the time, so no-one liked him and no-one could figure out why I was going out with him. But I became pregnant, and then my life just fell apart for about four or five years.

★ ★ ★

I came back to Sheffield to have this pregnancy terminated, and I had to see to it all myself. Colin, the bloke, wasn't of any help at all. In fact at the time when I realised I was pregnant Colin and I had split up and he was going out with somebody else. I had to ask the bank for an overdraft to pay for it and I lied saying it was for something else. And what stuck out in my brain when I went for this termination was that there was loads of other women and young girls there, but they all had somebody with them and I had no-one. Of all the times when I felt really isolated in my life, that was the worst.

This all happened in my two week holiday, then I went back to Brighton to continue with my training. I don't remember very much. All I know is that I couldn't see anybody, and all I did was cry. There was this really awful pain inside, a physical pain which totally immobilised me. I couldn't get off my bed. I felt sapped of energy, a complete wreck. I suppose I didn't want to do what I did, but I felt that it was the only thing I could do. I was such a bad person that I would make a horrible mother, so there was no way I could have this baby.

Our house warden, Mrs Averton, was really kind. She reminded me of my Grandma. She came and found me lying on the bed, and she said that people had been trying to knock on my door for about four days. Then the head of the school came, and the school tutor; I remember people flitting in and out. Then a consultant psychiatrist arrived from the local psychiatric hospital and he gave me some tablets that I didn't take. He asked if I would go to see him a couple of days later. I don't think I would have gone, but Mrs Averton came and took me in the car. He wanted to see me once a fortnight, but the next time I was supposed to see him I didn't turn up. I just started drinking really heavily – whisky. I hate whisky.

I stayed in my room all day and drank whisky and when it ran out I would go and get some more. That lasted for about four, five weeks – it was horrible – I was permanently drunk. Then I started to venture out of my room and I think that was when a lot of people became really concerned. So eventually I was admitted. The psychiatrist made it sound as if they were going to help me, and I think I recognised that I was totally out of control emotionally and that I had to do something. I went in voluntarily and I was in for about six weeks. They gave me tablets and I smoked 60 cigarettes a day. They referred me at some point to occupational therapy, where I could weave baskets if I wanted, or learn to type. I kept telling them that I *was* a typist and that I wasn't interested in weaving baskets, and their responses to that were, 'You're not trying to get better', so I went once and was bored to tears. I refused to go after that.

★ ★ ★

From my first admission to Basildon hospital onwards I was really un-controllably wild. I'd suppressed a whole lot of rage all my life and I think that the lid came off the anger. A lot of my rage came out when I was drunk – I had a lot of alcoholic black-outs – but I think one of the reasons I did drink so heavily was because it allowed me to get to a stage where I could get the anger out. I also started to cut myself again, only this time it was very badly. I have scars all over me where I had lots and lots of stitches. At one time I cut a vein or something – I lost a lot of blood. Almost always I was really drunk and I don't remember doing it, but on the very few occasions I do remember it didn't actually hurt at all. I think that when I've reached out for something to hurt myself with its been an absolute *pure* hatred of myself. I've found this really difficult to explain to other people because the idea of somebody cutting themselves is really odd and because sometimes people are quite horrified. Certainly the responses I've got from healthcare professionals when they've been stitching me up have been absolutely appalling. All they did was perpetuate what I already thought of myself with their attitudes. I've been told, 'Next time you do this, this is where you cut to kill yourself'. It's nothing to do with killing myself. I don't think I've ever had a gripe with life or living. I had a gripe with being me, which I found intolerable. I *hated* being me.

For the first couple of admissions I was diagnosed as suffering from depression. Nobody ever explained to me what that meant. I resigned from my nurse training because I couldn't cope with it, and the hospital admissions just escalated: it was literally in–out, in–out, for about four years altogether. Nothing ever happened; it was just a stream of different diagnoses that went from 'She's suffering from depression' to 'No, she's not suffering from depression, but she is depressed'. So there was a slight hiccup in the diagnostic process for a while, then eventually I was diagnosed as suffering from manic depression and I was told that this was an incurable illness.

Usually at this point I was sectioned, because I'd recognised after my second admission there that I didn't want to be there – that they weren't helping me – and I really hated the hospital, absolutely hated it. So every single admission, and there were many of them after that, I always ended up on either a section 2 or an emergency section (I think it's a section 5 or a section 4), and eventually I was locked up because I absconded. I hated that word, absconded. I've always associated it with being a criminal. I'd had so much of being bossed about and told what to do and when to do it: it was all about control. At this point I was constantly angry and they saw me as a difficult patient, a hateful patient even, and they got the full blast of my rage. Of course they saw that as a symptom of my illness.

I'd regularly stop taking the tablets in a fit of disgust, these don't work, and then be told, 'Well what do you expect? You're not going to feel any different if you don't take your tablets'. So I'd get into lulled into thinking 'Possibly they're right, I'll take the tablets again'. But I went through a whole stream of tablets. There was monoamine oxidase inhibitors, I had them for a while, overdosed on them and nearly killed myself. Lithium was probably the drug I've taken longest, because they convinced me what a marvellous wonder drug this was and definitely this was going to cure me. I took that for about eight or nine months and nothing happened. I narrowly escaped ECT, but I was regularly around people who were just zombified from ECT. Then the diagnosis changed again to personality disorder and then from personality disorder to borderline personality disorder, because they couldn't quite make up their minds. And with each diagnosis there was different set of medication, and then I ended up in a lock-up ward because I threw a paper cup at the dinner lady.

★ ★ ★

It went on my record that I was violent because I threw this paper cup – an empty paper cup by the way. I hadn't been eating for months, I'd lost lots and lots of weight, and my mum and dad had come down to visit me for the weekend. I'd had a row with my dad because he kept putting pressure on me to eat; in the end just to get them to leave me alone I agreed to go and eat. I went to this dinner lady and I'd missed the dinner time by about a minute and she screamed at me, 'You've already eaten!' Then my mum popped her head around the corner and just very politely said, 'You know she hasn't eaten anything, in fact she won't eat and we've just persuaded her'. 'Well she's too late', the dinner lady said – and she spoke to my mum as if she was a piece of dirt. Now bear in mind that I'd witnessed this dinner lady over and over again every single day for weeks and weeks talking to everybody as if they were nothing, it made me so angry that this anger just got overwhelming. It was a reflex kind of a thing that I threw this paper cup.

Not long after that I hit this male nurse who'd been continuously winding me up for quite a while. It started after I'd overdosed on the monos and I was unconscious for a couple of days. Apparently I was writhing around a lot and I didn't have any underwear on, just this hospital gown because I'd been transferred from the casualty department. When I'd been up and about for a few days, every time this male nurse was on duty he would make a point of making me feel really uncomfortable by very small sexual innuendos, 'Oh yeah, when you were unconscious you didn't have any knickers on'. Eventually, as I say, I hit him. I had no regrets about that at all. But when the consultant came the day my parents were brought down to be informed that I was being sent to a lock-up ward, he specifically asked me, 'How long have you been violent?' I said, 'I'm not violent', and that's how I got to know that this was all written down on my file. I was so angry. I'd actually explained all this to my consultant at Basildon and I thought that he'd listened and understood, but all that was down on my file was the dates and the times that I was violent, and this consultant regurgitated it. Within an hour or so I'd been packed off in an ambulance to Hopewell Hospital in Brighton, with my mum and dad tagging along in the car.

★ ★ ★

I stayed at Hopewell for a couple of months and I know the first week I was there I was totally in shock. *Totally* in shock. For them to send me here, these doctors who know what they are doing, I *must* be mad. They had a parole system so you couldn't go out, and you were literally locked in on a dormitory that ran into another dormitory and a lounge. Again nothing happened in terms of treatment, I was given more medication, Melleril, which is a mind-blowing, mind-bending horrible thing, you just can't hold your head up it's so heavy. It was a female ward, maybe 15 of us altogether, and a lot of the women had been transferred from C ward in Holloway Prison. I learned after a few weeks that a proportion of these women had committed really horrendous crimes – murders – and then I became even more angry. I hadn't done anything wrong, I hadn't hurt anybody, and here they were shoving me in this lock-up ward with people who'd murdered.

In a way it's very odd to describe being locked up as a positive experience, but in some respects it was. The good side of that was that I was forced to get to know these people. And when you listened to their life stories, in the same circumstances, I would have murdered as well. They'd been so badly beaten and abused over long, long periods that they'd responded in a very human way – they'd hit back. It had been very drastic and had resulted in murder, but I couldn't blame them. So that was a very positive experience that, knocked away a lot of stereotypes in my own head.

★ ★ ★

I can chuckle and think it's quite amusing now, but at the time it was absolutely horrific being locked up. You were all shoved in together so it didn't matter what your problems were or where you'd been or what your life had been like. You can imagine the most extreme forms of behaviour – bizarre and weird and frightening behaviour quite often – just flying all around you all the time. You become immune to it. You would sit there watching the telly and the next minute the telly would be picked up and thrown through the air by some disturbed patient and 'Oops there goes the telly', kind of thing. Or a patient might react to a nurse bossing them about by answering back and then a heated argument develops. It all gets out of hand literally within seconds, then the alarm buzzer would go and the next minute you'd just happen to turn around and there's maybe about five or ten nurses pinning someone down on the floor and injecting something like chlorpromazine up their bum. On maybe two or three occasions when I've really lost my temper: I've been pinned down and had injections of chlorpromazine, and there is nothing therapeutic in that, it's about ward control. I know sometimes I was obnoxious and hateful towards people, but more often than not it was provoked, in either discreet or indiscreet kinds of ways.

★ ★ ★

My dad died not long after I'd been discharged from the second admission to Hopewell. He had a stroke, but his heart was in an awful condition anyway so he didn't survive, and I think none of us really grieved. That sounds terrible, but it's just honest. For me it was a massive relief. Ever since I was a kid I'd always thought that had my mum died first I would have had to look after my dad, so that was part of it. I didn't go home: I went back to Brighton and was re-admitted and then I absconded. I think if I'd have had the psychological resources to withdraw myself entirely from the psychiatric system at that point I certainly would have done it, because I very much recognised that this wasn't helping me. I ended up back in the lock-up ward.

It was my third admission to Hopewell Hospital. I was told my section was to expire in two weeks time and the consultant wanted to replace it by a section 3. I said I wouldn't go to the bother of trying to get it lifted if it only had two weeks to run, I would stay voluntarily. I had nowhere that I wanted to be. I had a flat that they'd got me after my first admission and I hated it – it was always bombarded by other people. But no, he was absolutely adamant. His explanation for wanting to replace this section 2 by a section 3 was purely that I might be staying for a little while and there was no point in just repeating a section 2, but fortunately for me because I'd worked with people with mental handicap I was very much aware of what these sections were about and they certainly weren't there to be used by a psychiatrist just because it was convenient and less paper time for him. So I appealed and I got this section lifted, and not long after that I was transferred to an open ward and I just stayed put and became a good psychiatric patient in that I never challenged anything. Eventually I was referred to a clinical psychologist. I saw her for about a year and I think I spent the whole time just getting some of this anger out about my treatment in hospital.

★ ★ ★

After the third discharge from the Hopewell Hospital I went back to my flat and I started to do an Access course. Access courses are designed for mature students who haven't got formal qualifications to access higher education, so you do intensive study skills and modules of A-levels within a year or 18 months. I really enjoyed studying; I did an appreciation of art course within my Access course and I did a basic counselling course. I started to make sense of me a little bit in that course, though I'm surprised I finished it because I was still at this point not very well. Lianne, the clinical psychologist, negotiated an open ward policy for me, so rather than be dragged in kicking and screaming under a section I had to learn to go and ask for help, which I have always found really difficult anyway. I never made use of that because they never offered me any help as far as I was concerned. That was the last thing Lianne did and I was then allocated a social worker when she left.

The social worker was really, really nice. She listened to all my gripes and groans and moans and she suggested that I might benefit from this place called the Henderson Hospital. It's a therapeutic community for people with emotional problems. We arranged for an interview and I was accepted. It's quite a unique kind of place in that it's a National Health Service hospital, but the day-to-day work and control over the place is undertaken by the residents. The patients order the food and devise the menus; if anybody is distressed during the night they have a system whereby you'd be knocked up at 3 o'clock in the morning and you support one another throughout the night. It's totally no medication, so you weren't allowed to take medication unless it was for the physical side, and it was all based on therapy, group therapy. We had drama therapy, art therapy, and then small groups where you'd do more intimate, personal stuff. You'd have a communal meeting first thing, when the whole community would meet and discuss any problems with the group dynamics or whatever, and you'd have a work group as well. So in terms of the practical aspects of the running of the hospital the staff played a very minimal role, but in terms of therapy they were really skilled and very expert in their fields.

It was supposed to be for a maximum of a 12-month period, but I left after three months because it was just *so* overwhelming emotionally. I don't think I was in any way equipped to deal with groups and so many people. It was *really* hard work. The dynamics alone of living with 26 people were just *so* intense, all with their massive emotional problems. Lots of people self-harmed, lots of people had abused drugs or alcohol, so some would have bans. I had an alcohol ban so that meant I couldn't drink at all. There wasn't a person in there who I didn't warm to, because they had such sad stories to tell and they were so unbelievably supportive of one another. The biggest impact of the place for me was the drama therapy group. It was very very powerful, run by an extremely skilled man who was really good at his job. I think that was the first time I allowed myself to explore the stuff in my head. It was unbelievably painful. I just couldn't cope with it. So I went back to Brighton and finished my pre-Access course.

★ ★ ★

That little blast of the Henderson Hospital was just enough for me to know that if I worked really hard at it I could get my head sorted out. It wasn't the appropriate place for me to be – it was too overwhelming. But certainly it set me off in the right direction and I didn't take any medication from that point. I still got admitted to the hospital for being drunk or cutting myself or whatever, but I had regular contact with my social worker who was very supportive. She just said, 'OK it hasn't worked but we'll go on from here'. Then she gave me another good piece of advice. I told her that I was fed-up with thinking about my past: I didn't want to delve into the dynamics of my family, I just wanted to stop cutting myself and stop drinking and get on with my life. She got me an address for a rational emotive therapist in London, and I was in therapy with him for about four years.

Not long after I finished my Access course I came back to Sheffield. I applied to Sheffield Polytechnic to do my degree and was accepted onto that with my Access pass. I was going to pack in therapy and look for counselling services locally, but I'd got my head around this rational emotive therapy. It was very much about dealing with here and now, nothing like psychoanalysis when you explore childhood stuff, I didn't want to be bothered with any of that. So I continued, and all my therapy sessions were on the phone, which served a good purpose for me because I found face-to-face sessions particularly traumatic, because (a) it was a man, and (b) on the phone I could be personal in an impersonal kind of way.

Rational emotive therapy is not a regularly used technique in this country, it's very much American – a cousin in a way of cognitive behaviour therapy. It's not by any means a gentle therapeutic school of thought; it's very confrontative. The emphasis is on your faulty thought systems and not how you feel. But it did help, sort of. I don't think it was RET itself, but just the fact that for probably the first time in my life I stuck up for myself. It was really hard work because this man irritated me. I felt he was using me as a guinea pig, and I felt he was bossing me and that it was another form of brainwashing. His attitude was that if you learn the methods of RET it's like learning the ABC – you will be psychologically healthy – and that was a bit too simplistic for me.

But I persevered, and most of the hard work was the battles that I had with this therapist, because he had quite a strong personality and I felt overwhelmed by that at times. Saying that, he was very, very tolerant. I was really hard work myself. You know I would get drunk and be really abusive – and it embarrasses me to say that because I wouldn't dream of doing it now. It was just where I was at at the time, really deeply believing that I was bad and that this man was going to dump me any day. I think I tried to push him away. Sometimes I would ring up at 3 or 4 o'clock in the morning, drunk as a Lord, and he was practising from home so I would disturb his wife, drunk. I didn't put much thought into that, I was just so distressed. He was obnoxious too, but he stuck by me and no-one had ever really done that before. I really value that whole period.

★ ★ ★

I think the nicest day in my entire life was my graduation day. It was nothing to do with the award. I was pleased about that. It was just that I'd come so far from being a drunk and a seasoned loony, and there I was receiving my first class honours. My mum was there and my brother and my great aunt, it was a really lovely day. I couldn't believe I'd come so far when I know that lots and lots of people I was in hospital with are still wrapped up in that system, years on. I remember when I was in Hopewell once, they were having a sports day, and this psychiatric nurse really upset me because he asked me would I like to participate in the egg and spoon race. It was so patronising. I told him in not so polite terms where to shove his egg and his spoon and he wandered off, quite upset. I went over to a bench in the middle of this field somewhere and I sat there, sulking, and this lady came and sat next to me and said the usual kind of hospital thing, 'Got a fag?' Then she said, 'You're only a young girl, how old are you?' and I told her 26, and she said, 'I'm 62 now, I was 21 when I first started coming in here'. That's 40-odd years, isn't it, drifting in and out of the same place. God, I don't want that. So I haven't taken medication and I haven't been [back] in psychiatric hospital, though it was a struggle getting out of it. Now I do use RET, but I use it in my own way and not in a regimented kind of way. I'll pull out what is useful for me. What it's helped is that I'm so much calmer than I ever have been. I'm so interested and absorbed; there's a genuine interest in everything that I'm doing.

I drifted into social work, I think because most of my practical experience is in the care field. But the course was really gruelling. Eleven months out of the two years were placements, so they could send you anywhere, and consequently I had to move home four times within 18 months – that was really stressful in itself. And the academic side of it was so boring. Then more than anything I don't like social workers very much. I had a good experience with one social worker, but these people I trained with really irritated me: they did this all day long [*making scare quotes with the fingers of both hands*]. There were 32 people on our social work course, and 28 of them did this. And 'Ya, I hear what you're saying,' and 'Would you like to share with me?' They got on my nerves.

I chose not to practice; I chose to teach instead – mainly because I reckoned that I would never use my degree and I'd worked so hard for it. Now I'm lecturing part time at an FE college in health and social care, so I'm using my social work stuff all the time and my health studies degree, which I loved. I'm just applying to universities for lecturing positions, they're recruiting round about now for September, so we'll see how it goes. I really like teaching. I like the contact with the students. I've met really interesting people, and you *never* know what's coming up from day to day. I like the autonomy of lecturing as well. I get guidelines for the course and I mould it so it's mine.

Somebody rang me up the other day and asked me to talk to some mental healthcare managers. I know it would have to be different from the talks I would normally do in that they're so protective towards their professionality and would be intensely threatened by anything that was derogatory towards them. So I need to be really careful – not to watch what I say, I think I'm way beyond watching what I say about anything – but certainly to get a constructive message across. I really believe that unless professionals start relinquishing the power they have, or are even prepared to acknowledge that they hold that amount of power, then we're never going to get anywhere – and things aren't going to change.

PART THREE

Young men in crisis

8.

I'd rather it was a chapter I'd forgotten about: Paul Mann

From his deep voice on the telephone I was expecting a much older man, but Paul is surpisingly young when he answers the door. Neatly dressed in black jeans and a polo neck, he shows me to his room – a tiny add-on at the back of a 1930s semi where he lives with his mother and sister. It is packed from wall to ceiling with books, CDs and videos. Paul spends much of our talk referring to a series of typed notes marked 'Confidential'. This turns out to be a solicitor's report: he's in the process of suing the Health Authority for mismanagement of his case. The report cites a diagnosis of personality disorder, and the mismanagement in question is the inappropriate prescription of benzodiazepine tranquillisers.

I'm 22 and I live with my mother and sister. My father left home when I was eight, but I have remained in regular contact with him ever since. I had a reasonably normal and happy childhood. I attended the local high school and graduated at the age of 17 after doing a year in the sixth form.

Shortly after leaving school I had the notion of doing social work. Most of my family either work or have worked in the health service, my mother is a senior physiotherapist, my grandfather was a GP, my grandmother was a pharmacist, my father worked in a hospital even though formerly he was a computer teacher, so that quite appealed to me. I went on to college where I did a pre-social work course and took A-levels, which didn't go too well. I ended up with eight GCSEs and two A-levels in communication studies and sociology, both grades E.

During the course we had placements at all sorts of different places, and I quite fancied the idea of going into social work in the mental health field, because I'd had a placement at a hostel for the mentally ill. I was fascinated by the illness and the people; I wouldn't say it was fun, but it was stimulating. It was one day a week for a term. I used to take people out in the car and just sit and talk to them, and of course they've got great stories to tell. But at that stage I was quite a beginner to it.

Then I did a placement at the elderly people's home over the road, called The Everglades. Through the placement they offered me quite a lot of casual work while I was doing the course, and when I finished I went back there working as much relief time as I could. When a position became available they took me on full time. I quite liked the work, and they were fairly flexible hours. I got on very well with the residents and most of the staff. It's mainly a female environment as you can imagine, with it being care assistants and what have you. I was all right working with my colleagues, but when it came down to the supervisors I did have a few problems there, because obviously it was a bit of a step down from training for a career in social work to being a care assistant.

★ ★ ★

Things were going OK, but then in about May '93 I started having mild mood swings at work, which tended to be in the morning. The slightest thing could set me off; if I was criticised for a small thing I'd really take it personally and sink into a bit of a low. At other times I'd be quite unnaturally high, which didn't bother me too much. I didn't use to eat breakfast and I thought it was something to do with a lack of sugar in the morning – which could even have been the explanation. Later on the psychiatrist thought it might be manic depression [*laughing*]. Then there was the business of the probationary period when I was employed there. At the end of the six months, when I was starting to feel these mood swings and depression, they decided to extend the probationary period to nine months, which annoyed me a bit. After that it went up to 12, so they were prolonging it. But as you know employers can do that, and while you're on a probationary contract it's easier for them to dismiss you. I got to feel that I was being very unfairly treated.

I became depressed, well, as I said, I started to have low mood swings early in the morning. On one of these occasions Mrs Jarvis, my supervisor, came up to me and started remonstrating with me about a small and trivial item. I retaliated by saying that if I lost my job I'd probably go and kill myself. I meant what I said. Mrs Jarvis was very shocked and taken aback, and apparently she called an emergency meeting with my manageress, Mrs Hill, who came out of a meeting at another site to deal with the matter urgently. After that Mrs Hill spoke to me and suggested, or rather insisted, that I go to see my GP about the problem.

That was the first time in about 10 years I'd had contact with the GP, Dr Michaels. I'd never seen him before. He said he would like me to see a counsellor who was a community psychiatric nurse, so I said, 'Fine'. I saw her over a period of about eight weeks or so and it didn't really get anywhere. I think that was the first time I realised that I wasn't the sort of person that was susceptible to that kind of basic counselling for depression. I was only 19 or just 20. She did a lot of talking about psychotropic drugs and she went on about her own depression, which didn't help [laughs].

The doctor put me on paroxetine, one of the new SSRIs. That helped a little bit; what it tended to do was exaggerate the periods of elevation. But things at work were getting worse: the supervisor was being overcritical. Everything I did had to be reviewed, and I was so carefully monitored that it became unbearable in the end. But during this, I never displayed any of the symptoms to the residents: I was always professional with the people I worked with on the floor, so they had no problem with me.

★ ★ ★

The next chapter was a referral to a psychiatrist. The GP suggested I go because I'd been asking for Valium to supplement the antidepressant. I'd been feeling very anxious all the time for some while and he said, 'If you want that kind of thing, I'm going to get a proper diagnosis'. Now I was a bit dubious at first because of the stigma, but then I thought, 'Well, why not'. I got to feeling rather blasé – if they'd have offered me anything I would have taken it. I saw a registrar at Fairmount Hospital and he did a complete synopsis, or whatever you call it, and came up with a diagnosis of suspected bipolar disorder, which is pretty serious stuff. He doubled the antidepressants and said, 'See you in two weeks'.

At my next visit I was complaining about the anxiety and asking for something like Valium to supplement the antidepressants, because they can only do so much. He said, 'I'm not going to prescribe those because they're too addictive; let's try you on some haloperidol with procyclidine'. That was awful. I took it for about a week and it made me so apprehensive, shaky and restless, I literally couldn't keep still; it was doing the opposite to a tranquilliser. So I rang up my GP and he said, 'Stop taking it at once'.

Then one morning I was off sick and I was summoned to work for a meet-ing. The manageress was there with somebody from personnel and they said, 'We're very sorry but your probationary period is expired, we no longer want to keep you on'. I said, 'All right, fine', and later on that day I took an overdose of a combination of pills that I'd had stored up: the haloperidol, procyclidine, the antidepressants and some beta-blockers that had been prescribed – I was quite serious about it. But shortly afterwards, when I was lying there and these drugs were taking effect, I became very scared. I was thinking, 'What's going to happen? I might not die. I might just get cirrhosis of the liver or something' [*laughs*]. I thought, 'I don't really want to do this, I have a fear of pain'. I rang for the ambulance myself because there was nobody else about – my mother was in Devon, I don't know where my sister was. I was admitted that day I think. And because of the toxicity of the procyclidine, which is like atropine, it's very toxic, I was more or less out of it for the next couple of days, wander-ing around in a kind of psychotic haze, not knowing what I was doing. But when the effects of the drugs wore off I returned to normal.

★ ★ ★

It was a good kick start. I was quite anxious to get out of that acute ward. I only stayed there a week because when I came out of this drug-induced state I was quite perky. I asked to go and spend some time with my grandparents, which they agreed to. So I spent a week down in Somerset and my grandfather, who was a GP, suggested it might be a good idea if I saw the consultant rather than the registrar and got a proper diagnosis. He arranged for me to see the consultant privately because that was the only way of getting his time. So when I came back up north I went to see Dr Mainwaring, who said, 'Well, there is a possibility of manic depression. How about a trial of lithium?' I said, 'Fine'. I tried lithium for about a month, having all the nasty blood tests and things that went with it, and it didn't really do anything at all, so he said to stop taking it. I didn't get along that well with this consultant because I only saw him every two weeks or a month, and he'd just sit there for five minutes and say, 'How are you?' and 'OK, continue with the medication' or 'Let's try a new one'.

About that time I'd put in a complaint to the hospital about the prescrip-tion of haloperidol from the registrar, which my granddad had said was pretty out of order, and also about the waiting times to see the consultant. (After that first visit at the private hospital, he'd said, 'Come back and see me on the

NHS, it'll be easier that way'.) Anyway, this complaint was basically just dismissed, which I felt a bit bitter about.

Then in January '94 I saw the senior house officer because the consultant was away. He took me off the antidepressant and put me on a fairly high dose of sertraline. The next month I saw Dr Mainwaring again and this time I was wanting more drugs to try and combat symptoms. I'd asked for Stelazine, which he gave me – basically I was just desperate for anything that would alleviate things. He also referred me to a psychologist up at the hospital, Vivien Brice, who I saw for cognitive behaviour therapy. That didn't really work either. To be honest it came across as very simplistic; I'd just done an A-level in psychology at college and this was all old hat.

★ ★ ★

At my first meeting with Ms Brice she'd asked me to fill out work sheets to show how I was feeling on an hour-by-hour basis during the day, and I'd filled these out over a period of three weeks in between my first and second appointments.

Unfortunately on the second visit, with these highs I'd been having and these fantasies of grandeur, I'd dressed up in a doctor's coat. It was more as a joke than anything serious – I think maybe out of boredom – but obviously she was a bit concerned. This all sounds very silly to me reading it off: I'd rather it was a chapter I'd forgotten about.

I'd filled out these work sheets. I was perfectly honest about everything as I was meant to be. One day I felt particularly angry at Dr Mainwaring because my complaints against him had been dismissed by the hospital and because his treatment of me did not seem to be making things any better. I put on the form, 'Felt like shooting Dr Mainwaring', not that I was going to do it, that was only a passing thought – I mean I hadn't even got a gun – but I was quite angry with him for having dismissed these complaints and I thought I was getting a bit of a sloppy service. I also told her that I'd carried a knife to one of my sessions with my GP and the psychiatrist, because I was desperate for somebody to prescribe me Valium, which by now I saw as being the be-all-and-end-all, the shining star, the ultimate cure for the anxiety and what have you, and nobody was prepared to prescribe it because they said it was too addictive. I said I was going to, not threaten them, but say, 'Give me the Valium or else', kind of thing, though I never actually produced a knife, it was just a thought. All the time in the back of my mind I knew it was not really a wise thing to do, and I was also calling myself doctor at the time with the fantasy of being a PhD in psychology, because I'd read up about the subject, and obviously to a psychologist this looks like bad news. Anyway she reported me to the GP, the consultant, and the police. This was without telling me. I mean she told me that she had reported it to my GP and Dr Mainwaring, but she didn't give me any indication of how seriously she took this comment about shooting Dr Mainwaring. I could understand her concern – I mean I could have been a psychopath – but she could have taken the time to question me further as to whether it was a joke or a serious threat and I was going to go out and buy a .45 or something.

So, third meeting with Ms Brice, went OK, wasn't dressed as a doctor that time, but she decided to terminate the meetings because the therapy was going nowhere.   ✦

★ ★ ★

About a week later I went to see a friend of mine who was an inpatient on one of the wards at Fairmount. As a joke I put on the white coat with the badge and when I got to the door there were two policemen there. At first I thought they must be there for another incident, because the glass had been broken on one of the doors. So I was minding my own business, head down, just going past them. I didn't realise they were there to intercept me, because I couldn't think who'd phone the police and say I was going there. I think I know who it was now. I won't mention her name because she's a friend of mine, and I think it was more out of concern for me than any overzealousness on her part. Well, the police expected me to be carrying a knife or something, which I wasn't – they searched me – and I said I was going to see an old friend, maybe they interpreted that as being Dr Mainwaring. Obviously they asked me about the badge, which looked a bit suspect, even though it wasn't inferring I was a doctor of medicine, it just said PhD in psychology, with a photo on – they took that seriously. They'd heard about these threats with the knife, alleged threats, and so they detained me under section 136 of the Mental Health Act and took me down to the police station.

Normally you're supposed to be seen by your own GP and psychiatrist if possible. But neither of them were available, so I was seen first by the police surgeon, he always sees you separately. He asked me questions like, 'Do you know what you're doing?' and 'Why are you doing this?' and 'Who are you?' I only spent about five minutes with him, just rationalising the situation, saying this has been taken out of proportion. About five hours later the multidisciplinary team arrived, made up of a consultant psychiatrist from Fairmount and two approved social workers. A solicitor was there as well, but he didn't actually do anything, in fact he assisted the multi-disciplinary team more than defend me. It was an unusual situation: I wasn't, for some reason, really frightened about sitting and talking to them; it had got to the stage where I wasn't that bothered – I was feeling quite well, quite high even – but ultimately I did end up saying a few things that would have come across as odd, about these fantasies of being a doctor and what have you. And because of the alleged threats they put me under a section 2, even though I'd stipulated that I'd be quite happy to go in as a voluntary patient because I felt the need for a few weeks in hospital just to put a lid on things. In fact I'd mentioned this about a month before to the consultant, Dr Mainwaring, and he'd said, 'No'. So, in a way, during that multidisciplinary team meeting, it was partly my intention to try and get myself admitted. The solicitor said to me, 'I know you've asked to go in as a voluntary patient, but the police have insisted that you are sectioned, otherwise they will press charges themselves for impersonating a doctor, so it's best to go down, as the social worker put it, the social worker route'. Which I suppose it was. But because of the problems at Fairmount, they thought it best if I was taken to a secure ward in Maidlow Hospital, that's a psychiatric hospital about 20 miles away.

Before I was arrested and admitted I'd been to see my GP and complained to him about my condition following the termination of the cognitive behavioural therapy with Ms Brice. I was beginning to feel more agitated. On previous occasions Dr Michaels had always said that he would never put me on Valium because it was so addictive. But at our meeting in March he prescribed me 5 mg of diazepam twice a day.

★ ★ ★

Well, Maidlow Hospital was certainly more modern than Fairmount, but it was rough in the sense that there were a lot of potentially quite violent people on that ward. There were quite often outbursts of aggression, from the staff as well, which I didn't think I'd see after the 1984 Mental Health Act. It wasn't that widespread, it was mainly one member of staff who got a little bit physical with one or two of the patients who were causing an uproar, which was wrong of him. I did witness him physically abusing one of the female patients, lifting her up off the ground and running and forcing her against a window. He was a big bloke, he just lost his rag and grabbed her up off the floor screaming and swearing at him. Everyone was quite aware of it, the staff accepted it, the patients had to put up with it. So in that sense it was a little uncomfortable, but I soon got used to it and made a few friends there, and the staff accepted me as being, like, the perfect patient. They'd say wish they were all like me and that. I think everyone wondered what I was doing there. In fact, it took quite a bit of convincing one of the female patients that I was a patient and not some sort of spy.

While I was in there I was seen by a consultant registrar who came up with a whole list of possibilities. The feeling I got was that psychiatrists, especially young ambitious ones, aren't happy unless they've found a label for somebody, and this was puzzling them. They'd gone to the trouble of sectioning me, and for them to turn around and say, 'There's nothing really wrong with you' insults their pride really. So a couple of weeks later I was seen by a forensic consultant psychiatrist called Dr Bushnell, a very good doctor. He made about three or four lengthy visits, and he came up with quite a long report for the tribunal, because obviously I'd appealed against the section 2. The report basically said that there was a possibility of either a developing schizoid illness, an organic brain disorder, or a personality disorder – which is the one he went for. He actually said in this report, 'I can't see any reason for keeping this man in', but on the evidence of the ambitious registrar and the RMO who was my consultant at the ward, the tribunal decided, 'Well it's only a section 2, he might as well stay here for the rest of the two weeks'. I'm very thankful for seeing Dr Bushnell because he was the most perceptive and understanding doctor, the first doctor who I felt knew what he was talking about – who was listening to me and made an accurate diagnosis of what was wrong.

★ ★ ★

When I was admitted I was taken off most of the medication and just left on the antidepressants, and apart from the side effects of coming off diazepam and beta-blockers, the increased anxiety, I think it probably made me feel better. I was so bogged down with all these pills, it was possibly why I'd got into so much trouble in the first place. Everything went fine, and at the end of it the RMO [resident medical officer] said, 'Legally we can't keep you in here', and I was released. They said they'd arrange a CPN [community psychiatric nurse] for me, but she never showed up because she came under the Fairmount jurisdiction where I'd had all the trouble, and they were refusing any more referrals or treatment. So I couldn't have a CPN, I wasn't allowed to see any of their psychiatrists, and I was left basically with no back-up.

So I went back to see my GP, Dr Michaels, and he put me back on the diazepam and gave me amitripytline as well, which is a tricyclic antidepressant. But by this time the diazepam was causing drowsiness and difficulty in concentrating, and it was affecting my sleep as well – I found that I couldn't sleep without it, and with it I didn't sleep that well – so it really was interrupting things, and I had low blood pressure ... [*leafing through notes*]. In July he changed the diazepam tablets for diazepam syrup, then in August, changed the syrup for temazepam, which is a sleeping tablet, by which time I was getting higher and higher dosages. At that meeting Dr Michaels was getting a bit sick of me, and he threatened to take me off his list because he said I was too much trouble. Bear in mind at this time that I'd had to find my own social worker, because I wasn't assigned one; he refused a CPN, and he refused referrals to the psychiatric team, so I was basically just left with him. I'd also asked him to support my application for housing, which he said he'd do, but he never got around to it.

Before he took me off his list I decided, 'Right, I'm going to leave anyway, go to a different practice'. I consulted a solicitor about it, and he reckoned we could bring a case against Dr Michaels for prescribing diazepam over a period of time to somebody of my age, even though every other psychiatrist and doctor had said no, it's too addictive. I admit I had been asking for it, but that's no reason to prescribe it just because a patient wants it. Basically I didn't realise and he didn't tell me about the side-effects: the sleep fluctuations, drowsiness, and the lack of coordination; it was slowing me down and affecting my weight as well. I mean it's a wonderful drug in the short-term, it does make things feel a lot better, but you just need more and more and when you try and come off it just doubles the symptoms. That's why it's rarely prescribed nowadays. In fact my grandfather told me that he'd rarely prescribed it and if patients insisted he'd ask them to sign a disclaimer saying they wouldn't sue him, and he'd retired seven years previously. He thought it was disgusting. Interestingly enough, Dr Michaels had said months and months before, when I was first seeing him, that he never prescribed it at all. Yet here he was prescribing it to me quite happily because he was just so eager to pass me off with a drug rather than spend time with me.

★ ★ ★

After I'd left Dr Michaels and joined the new practice, the doctor there took me off the Valium and I was just left on the antidepressant. So the case has been going on and is still going on today. I'm sending off all these medical notes to an expert for assessment, then the Legal Aid will either say yes or no to taking it to court, and then it's up to the medical expert, whether or not he thinks it's medical negligence in the first place.

After I'd been refused any more treatment at Fairmount, I saw an advert for a private psychotherapy practice and I thought I'd give it a try. This private psychotherapist was very good. I only saw her once, though it was quite a long session. She was into regressive therapy – childhood and all that – and hypnosis. It was positive and encouraging. Here she was, a non-medical person, not interested in drugs or anything like that, but into relaxation. It was like a breath of fresh air. But I couldn't afford to keep going, so I asked the new GP whether they could pay for it, because I found it much more beneficial than seeing a psychiatrist, and they said no, but they would refer me to their own psychologist. I've not as yet seen him, apparently they're setting up a referral and it takes a long time. I wish they'd hurry up about it.

I managed to wean myself off the temazepam and diazepam. Well the craving's still there, every time I feel anxious I know that a Valium would just make it disappear, but I haven't got that luxury anymore. I just have to cope with it in other ways. And recently I was in America – my grandmother was going over to the States to visit my aunt who lives in California and she asked if I'd like to go with her as a twenty-first birthday present, so I jumped at the chance – that was November last year. While I was over there I ran out of the antidepressants, so I thought that would be a good time to stop taking them as well. So in actual fact at the moment I'm on no medication at all. The doctor is still signing me off sick, but its getting to the stage where she's saying she can't really justify it much longer, even though I don't feel up to working.

At the moment I'm doing this Open University course in psychology. It'll take me five or six years to qualify so that means I can't be doing a full-time job. It's very hard getting back into the swing of writing essays and disciplining myself. It will take a lot of perseverance. In the end there's a slim chance of becoming a clinical psychologist. It sounds very nice and its something I'm interested in, but I'm not exactly optimistic about becoming one. Then there's the voluntary work, driving mainly, and I've offered my services to Mind, but I think sometime in the future I'll have to find some sort of paid employment. I'm getting towards becoming ready for that kind of thing. I'm fortunate in that I've got a good GP. I'm hoping this psychology referral comes through, and I'm hoping to get independent accommodation. Somebody from the council is coming to see me tomorrow. I do realise that there's a lot more needy people in front of me, but it is detrimental to my health to stay here because of the bad relations with my mother and my sister, and I need more space.

★ ★ ★

I can read you this. It's actually a report from the solicitor, basically like what you're doing. He taped it and then typed it up, the history of my case. 'So to sum up', like I've said, 'since I've withdrawn from the drugs and had the psychotherapy which involves some hypnosis and regression together with relaxation it has focused my mind on the real cause of my problems. It is true to say that I now realise that the stress at work brought to the surface problems that have been deep rooted and in my subconscious for many years. It was not until I had the hypnosis and was told the result of it that I was able to focus on what was causing my mental condition. Since then I've been able to work on that problem in a positive way. I still need, however, further treatments of psychotherapy, and I am hoping to have it funded by my GP. I now realise that over the last 15 months I've been prescribed various chemicals which have sent me in ever-decreasing circles. I have languished in a drug-influenced environment. The fact is that the various drugs have not cured me, have increased my mistrust of doctors and heightened my anxiety. Since I've come off the drugs I've done various things to occupy myself. I have tried to start a video business for weddings and birthdays; I have started an Open University degree course in psychology; I've become actively involved in photography and in keeping animals at home; I am actively engaged in seeking out my own accommodation; I am seeking voluntary work. All the above has occupied my time and stopped me becoming introspective. The psychotherapy helped me do all these things, but once again I need it to continue in order to get fully better'.

9.

Doing all right, considering: Adrian Stiles

I met Adrian at his house, a one-up one-down terrace on a new estate, where he lives on his own. He's a big man in his late 30s, with a shy, withdrawn manner and a quiet voice, often trailing off into silence. He works as a computer programmer. He was a postgraduate researcher when he had his first breakdown, following a serious crush on a female fellow student who did not return his affections.

I come from a small village in the Midlands and I went to a local school. My father ran a road haulage business. My mother stayed home as a housewife, she was very quiet and very loving. When I left school I joined a bank. You know how it is when you're young, you don't want to spend 50 years in a bank, so I gave that up and went to the college of further education. I got four 'A's and went to Leeds University to do mathematics. The first year there I had a shared room in digs. I found it difficult to make friends, but I made one or two. We used to play cards or go to the pub. So I did three years there and then got a First. No problems there.

I wanted to do post-grad, and I was offered a good place to stay on where I was, but I thought I'd go for a change. I eventually plumped for a university near to where my parents lived, where I grew up, and I got a three-year grant. It was MSc, then go on to a PhD.

The course work at this new place was very difficult because it was advanced from where I'd been, so I was a bit disheartened. In fact a girl came down from my previous university the same time as me, and she got completely stuck and gave it up and went back, but I plodded on.

I was living in a block of flats on campus with about 12 postgraduates. That was quite strange. I hid away in my room most of the time. And somehow I met Sofia…she took an interest in me or made a play for me or something.

We used to walk back from lectures and have coffee in each other's rooms. She was into schizophrenia and she used to say that mental patients were mistreated in hospital and that they were stripped, prodded and herded around like elephants, to use her words. And she was a mystery, you know? I can't explain it. I'd never had that close friendship with a pretty lady before, so it was very special to me that this friendship with her should go right. It lasted for a term. At the end of the first term I was hit by an arrow. I know this sounds strange, but I really was. My heart exploded, I was completely overwhelmed, and it lead to one thing and another. I was coolly rejected by Sofia, and this caused me great pain and great anxiety. I was very distraught. I went home for Christmas afterwards, and when I came back I tried to get on with the work again, but I was too distracted.

★ ★ ★

So the second term I just went to lectures. I was completely distraught and I suppose I was isolated, I hadn't made any other friendships really. And I couldn't stay where I was, I was pining away; I lost a lot of weight, several stone probably. So I went on holiday, but I was completely mixed up. Then I saw Sofia again, which was a mistake because she was very nasty in the end...and as a result of this I couldn't do my work anymore, I'd lost the ability and how was I going to cope? I didn't know that doctors had drugs that could have mended that, I thought there was no cure. I was misled by reading Laing actually, because he suggests it's a journey you go through and you come out the other side. I think now it is an illness and you actually need the drugs to alleviate the symptoms. But I didn't think that then.

I saw the tutor at my first university and transferred back. I ended up in a bedsit, and I ended up seeing the admissions tutor again and I said to him, 'Look, I've gone nuts'; for some reason I trusted him with this information. So I ended up going back there as a pretend student; they'd taken me on as a student, but what I was doing I don't bloody know because I couldn't think straight. This tutor obviously didn't realise how distraught I was. He gave me the address of some people who did co-counselling and I went round to them but we didn't mesh, so I didn't get any further with that. And eventually after a few months he suggested I go to the student health service. So I did that, and of course I said I couldn't work or something; I didn't explain it very well. I had some ideas, but I was integrating my heart in a way, integrating a lot of emotion and stuff that I wasn't normally aware of. I was a bit mixed up, but I knew what I was doing and I needed someone I could talk to, someone more on my level. Anyway, the doctor said, 'Come back in two weeks'. That was it. Well I felt pretty hopeless. Things got out of hand. And at Christmas time I gave up the bedsitter and went home.

Yeah, I went back home and then a letter arrived saying I needed a doctor's certificate, so I ended up calling the doctor – he'd been the family GP since I was little. He came to the house to see me, but he didn't say much and I didn't say much; I think my father did all the talking. Then there was an appointment with the psychiatrist and my father took me there, we parked a long way away so we had to walk. I went and saw this guy and he'd got himself behind the desk in a big chair and I sat in this squadgy chair opposite, and I made some allusions to Wagner's *Ring* and other things, and he didn't get them, he just said, hmmm, he wanted to speak to my father. I didn't speak to him for more than two minutes. I went down, got my father and waited downstairs and then came back up again and he said, 'It's something that happens to intelligent people, their thinking becomes muddled.' He said, 'Come into hospital for two weeks and then go back to university and how about that?' I thought well, I'll settle with that.

★ ★ ★

I had no idea at all what hospital would be like. I imagined it'd be a place where you could rest in peace and quiet and you'd have people to talk to about your problems and they'd help you sort things out. But it wasn't to be. I tried to talk about all the things that had been going on when I first saw a doctor, but she gave no response. No-one ever gave me any feedback or response. I think they got the wrong idea entirely, from the beginning. They had no idea of my real problem, I'm sure of that. They were just going to clear it up. Yes, that's what the doctor in the first interview said, 'We'll soon clear this up.'

The next day they sent me down to this place somewhere, put me on a couch, and gave me this form to sign. It said something about electroplexy, and I didn't know what it meant, I had no idea, I was just going along with them. It's very difficult to say 'No' when you're the sort of person who tends to conform and go along with people. I mean, my opinion now for anyone who's offered ECT is 'Just say no', as they say. And ask for a second opinion... ECT destroyed my intellect. I was reduced from someone who was always inspired by this love to sitting with these people sticking little squares in a tray.

I was desperate to sort out these problems. They didn't sort out the problems, they *removed* them: they removed my *knowledge* of them.

I had 12 ECTs so I must have been in there for some time, but I don't remember much about it. Well, I remember the first time because they showed me the form. I remember they'd come and stick a thing in the back of your hand where they'd do the anaesthetic or whatever. I remember the last one because she came out and said, 'Make the most of it, it's your last'. And I remember one in the middle when I had this terrible experience where I couldn't breathe – I was lying there unable to move, unable to breathe and still conscious, and I was absolutely terrified until I passed out. That's about all I remember.

★ ★ ★

I stayed at home 'til the autumn term came round. Then I went back to university, studied a new topic with a different tutor, and picked up from scratch. In a way it was as well I went home and things were reconciled with the family, because there was difficulties there in that I was trying to be myself, and it came to a head with this Sofia stuff. There were things Sofia had fed in, she was completely poisonous…she really was. But it was really difficult. I'd lost my ability, my skill at my work, and I didn't know whether there was any way of getting it back. And I found that without that there was very little I could do – I was completely lost. There's a feeling of numbness, still; things don't flow like they used to.

I became very angry about this ECT, because I was looking up what it was and what had been done. I went round to the co-counselling people the admissions tutor had introduced me to and started doing that, but it was just trying to sort things out after the event. It was too late after, because I no longer had the feelings; I'd lost the emotional content. I mean I'd absolutely worshipped Sofia. I even once offered to be her slave [*laughs*], so I was completely crushed by it. I'd lost a lot, but I'd also gained a lot, if you can understand that. I'd gained this great emotional awareness, and then the ECT took away the inspiration. I was really reduced to square zero.

I suppose I slowly put things together, and did the co-counselling and got the PhD. My mother died just before that. At the end I was still very disturbed about this ECT business. That was how I came to get involved again, because I got scarlet fever after I'd finished university, so I saw the GP, and it was then I started complaining about the ECT and about what they'd done to me. And he referred me to a psychiatrist and the psychiatrist said he would see me and let me talk to him about things, but again it was *too* late, it was *after* the event and there's nothing you can do afterwards, nobody can do anything about it once it's been done.

★ ★ ★

I got offered a job after I got my PhD, but because of this feeling I had after the ECT, I didn't take it on. I remained in Leeds and stayed with some people I'd met doing co-counselling, then took on a part-time MSc. I didn't know what else to do really. I got half way through that and then I had a different sort of breakdown, and I left and went home. But it wasn't much of a home to go to now: as I say my mother had died in '79; my father had made house with this other woman, and at the time this breakdown occurred he'd fallen out with this other woman and he was lodging somewhere. But my brother was there and he put me up. I went to the GP and all I got from him was, 'What sort of drugs are you on? What sort of drugs do you take?' I couldn't believe the hassle. He said he'd make an appointment for me with a psychiatrist. But before that things were getting out of hand.

My brother took me to Leamington and put me in a bed and breakfast. I didn't want to stay in this bed and breakfast, so I got my things and went out, and I was going down the street into town when I was stopped by a policeman and a policewoman, who wanted to know what was in my suitcase. Well eventually they looked in my suitcase, and then I carried on and found a hotel. I got a room in this hotel, but they'd got some sort of noisy party going on so I went out again. I had my key with me and there was this guy on the door. I said, 'Do you want me to leave the key or shall I take it with me?' And he took the key out of my hand, took it away. So the next time I wanted to go out, I went down the fire exit instead of going past this guy, and there was no way out, it was completely dark, I had to come back in and it ended up with the police being called and me being taken to the station. They called my father and my brother, who picked me up and took me home, and the psychiatrist came out on a Sunday.

The next day I went into hospital in Coventry on a section. They wanted me in my pyjamas so they could examine me, then they hid my clothes so I couldn't escape. Nobody was particularly helpful in this hospital. After a couple of weeks they came round saying that I wouldn't need breakfast that morning because I was having some treatment, and I knew that meant ECT because they don't give you breakfast if they're giving you ECT. So I said, 'I'm not having that'. And it was mysterious, they brought some guy to talk to me in the common room, I don't know whether he was another doctor or what he was. Then a day later, a *gang* of male nurses came into the room with an injection, and I said were they going to force me to have that and they said they were. So I obviously couldn't do much about it and let them do it. I can only assume it was because they didn't like me refusing the ECT. I was no trouble at all. It was Depixol. I've had it for 10 years now. Maybe it was the right stuff – I mean, it probably works, but the tablets were working anyway and the way they came and gave it me, really. I'm really angry about it.

★ ★ ★

I suppose I must have stayed there another two weeks. They wanted me to have another injection before they let me out, so eventually I let them give me another injection, but I was so angry about the way I'd been treated that…well, I moved to Guildford. I'd had some friends there when I was doing my PhD, so I'd got to know it. The psychiatrist thought I'd gone to get out of his jurisdiction. His only reason for giving me an injection was that he could use a smaller dose, so he said. But anyway, this didn't completely clear up the problem and I ended up going back to Leeds. I went to the GP in Leeds, and he referred me back to the psychiatrist who suggested coming into hospital. Of course I wasn't in such a state then because the drugs had relieved my anxiety so I could relax a bit and take it easy, and that's what I did. I went into the Northern General and had a reasonably pleasant summer.

They kept me on the Depixol – they reckoned it was all that was keeping me well – and I made friends with this manic girl who turned out to be a very good friend. I was a bit worried to start with because I was sitting watching television and she came and sat behind me and started whispering, 'There's nothing wrong with you' [*laughing*], and then she started talking about Dada and Dali – she was high, you know. I thought, 'This is a very strange girl here', but she was very nice, she was an architecture student in London. She'd gone manic and been in hospital in London, and had somehow come back home to Leeds and gone to hospital there. They brought her down from her mania but she was never quite straight… [*laughs*] – she was very nice. She got me a little job doing some programming on her father's pocket calculator when I left. He's a hinge manufacturer and er, I did this little programming job for her [*laughs*]. That made it a pleasant stay actually.

★ ★ ★

I restarted my MSc course half way through and finished that, still having the Depixol. Then I got a job down in Wiltshire, doing research for the forestry commission. It was nice research: computer statistics. I went to Wales a couple of times and dug some boreholes. I did that for about a year.

Then I told my GP I was going to stop taking the Depixol, I'd been having it for years, and I eventually said I'm not having any more. But a few months later all the worries that had caused the second breakdown started overwhelming me again, and I ended up going into a psychiatric ward in a general hospital in Wiltshire. I suppose that was an escape really. There were a couple of nurses there who were quite friendly. I didn't take part in the day-to-day activities, the occupational therapy and stuff like that, I didn't do that until much later when they sent me to the day centre. I don't know what to say about it really. I was bothered they were giving me too much drugs, they were giving me much higher doses than I'd had and I wasn't happy about that. But *they* said it was all right, you know, and they were quite good. We even had some little groups in people's houses. I was there six months, though it didn't seem that long at the time. Again there wasn't much in terms of counselling or talking about your problems. It was just somewhere safe to stay. I used to go into the village, walk round and walk back again to the hospital.

★ ★ ★

After I left I started my research job again and began looking around for other work, as that was temporary, and after a few months I found this job round here. Luckily they didn't ask too many questions. I got this job as an analyst programmer, found a bedsitter, and continued having the Depixol. I've been here since '86, in this house since '88. Every couple of years I seem to have some sort of setback. I've been in hospital once, 1990 probably. I'm on Stelazine tablets and Depixol injections every two weeks, 40 mg. I was on 100 mg of Depixol in the hospital in Wiltshire, and they got it back down to 40 mg when I came here.

I think I've got used to having the drugs. I was never happy about it at first, I always wanted to stop taking them as soon as I started, but it seems to hold things together. It stops you getting stuck in crap, where everything becomes significant and everything becomes personal, where you read too much into things, well that's what happens to me anyway. Essentially I can't do anything when I'm in that state. And it takes a while to get back to normal again, a month or so. It's not an instant, overnight changing back to normal, it has to work itself out somehow.

I suppose I'm doing all right, considering all the problems, but it's taken a long time, with a lot of setbacks on the way. I think I've got a wider perspective just growing older, I look at things in a different way really. I got into great knots after Sofia. Great knots about how other people saw me, how other people were different with different value systems, the whole thing. I'm not so bothered now about these things, but they seemed desperately important at the time. I suppose it's probably the drugs, but I've also relaxed into myself... a bit too relaxed probably.

The boss threatened to sack me not so long ago. For some time I'd been fairly lax in my time keeping and I hadn't been doing quite the hours, and then my father was really ill. He'd had this operation for cancer and he'd come home and then he had some sort of stroke; he was suddenly taken very ill and taken back into hospital. So I went off one afternoon to visit him and left a message at work to say where I was going and that I'd ring around lunchtime. And before lunchtime I got a phone call from the boss, which was really awkward, and then he started sending me endless letters saying that I was going to be sacked. I just took a couple of months off because I couldn't cope with this ...I had to see my father. If the trouble hadn't blown up at work maybe I could have kept on trying to do both, but with all the trouble I didn't know what was going on. When I went back to work he wanted me to sign this big document saying that if I had a day off or came late I was going to be sacked. I was a bit iffy about signing this document and that created another disturbance, but I eventually signed it.

I hope to move on to something else before too long. I'd quite like to go back home now. My thought would be to work with my brothers in the family business, they run a garage. Maybe some day.

10.

It does teach you a bit about human nature: Graeme Wilson

Graeme came to see me one weekend when he was visiting a cousin of his in my neighbourhood. He's bright, youngish looking, probably in his mid-30s, tall and slim, and his conversation is animated. For the past few years he's been doing voluntary work as a software consultant and mental health trainer. He started by showing me some laminated guides, 'Dealing with the Mentally Ill', which he produced for the Metropolitan Police. Graeme was hospitalised for six years, on and off, with a diagnosis of schizophrenia, and then he spent as long again as an outpatient, though you would never know it. He stopped taking medication two years ago.

I got ill at university, when I was 20. I took a year off after school and went to India for four months, then came back and I had a job in a local multistorey car park. That was a really good job, fascinating. I went to Leicester University in October 1979 and got ill two weeks into the summer term. The first thing that happened was that I would start going to lectures that weren't my lectures, so I'd turn up to an engineering lecture or a physics lecture or something and I'd understand everything that was said at the lecture. I was actually reading French so that was a bit weird. That came first, and then I started hearing voices, and they said pretty much the sort of things that I said in that sheet – that I was a useless shit and I should kill myself and if I didn't kill myself then they would. I didn't think about the logic of that, I just accepted it. Certainly to begin with I don't think I found it particularly distressing, which sounds strange in view of what they were saying, but later I think I was slightly high, and things became very strange.

At that time Leicester had a system of personal tutors. Everyone had a personal tutor in a hall who was in theory supposed to look after people's personal welfare. I never actually met mine, as far as I know I don't think anybody met him. Presumably they did by coincidence, but there was never any organised attempt as far as I'm aware for hall tutors to meet the students. And in fact the only two people who took an interest were the Anglican chaplain at the university – I'd started going to Anglican church services as well, which was very out of character – and the hall warden. In the end the hall warden phoned my parents and they came and fetched me back from Leicester and I spent some months back home, which was probably more difficult for my parents than it was for me, because I kept wandering off. Sometimes I would just wander around where I lived – I'd go 10, 20 miles – and sometimes I'd go walkabout. I went up to Nottingham on one occasion; I was picked up by the police and my parents had to drive up and bring me back. The police were very good, the police have always been very good. I think that's the general experience of most people I've come across; they don't mind the police because the police admit they don't know much about that and they don't try and pretend they do. Anyway, I was persuaded to go and see my GP, and my GP said that I ought to go and see a psychiatrist, and several weeks later I agreed to that. So I did see a psychiatrist, saw him privately twice, and then he said I should go into hospital, but he also said that there wasn't much point in going to him privately because it was very expensive, and that the only thing that would be better if I'd stay privately would be the food, and I think he was probably right. I went into Fairfield, which is one of a cluster of hospitals around Weybridge. There used to be five or six and most of them have been closed down now. I went into Fairfield, I think, in October 1980 and was there on and off for the next five, six years.

When I first went to see the psychiatrist he put me onto a very low dose of Depixol, an antidepressant dose. As you know, Depixol if you give it in high doses is an antipsychotic, and in very low doses is an antidepressant. And given that there are lots of other antidepressants that he could have chosen, it's interesting that he chose that one. I never really discussed it with him, but it seems a possibility that he suspected even at that stage that there was slightly more to it than just depression. All that happened when I went into hospital was they just whacked up the dose as double injections; I wasn't particularly sedated or anything. Then he decided to change tack and I went onto Largactil, slightly over the maximum recommended dose. The Royal College has a wonderful euphemism for that: a dose above the maximum recommended dose is a high dose, it's not an excessively high dose, but it's a high dose, according to the Royal College. After that most of the time actually I was on Largactil – no I wasn't, because it caused sunburn: during the summer I'd go onto Melleril and during the winter I'd go back to Largactil, so my prescription was seasonal.

★ ★ ★

I was in a rather unfortunate position because I didn't suffer too much from side-effects, well visible side-effects; my hands didn't shake too much. My speech was a bit slurred, but the side-effects weren't a terrific problem, though sometimes there was acute dystonic reactions: my arms would suddenly go weird and get forced behind my head and get fixed there, as if I was asking a question all the time, and my neck would seize up and go back or forward or go down, so I needed a jab of Kemadrin occasionally, and that got rid of those side-effects. But the trouble was, because I had fairly few problems from side-effects, the doctors felt able to push the dose up really high, and one of the drugs I was on at one stage, pimozide, causes heart damage: it killed 11 or 13 people in this country prior to 1990. I'm not sure whether it killed them over a long period of time and suddenly somebody twigged that it was the pills that were doing it, or whether they all died within a very short period, but anyway, in November 1990, I think it was, my psychiatrist actually rang me up and said, 'Are you still taking the pimozide?' I said, 'Yes', and he said, 'Well don't'. He was forthright, he didn't mince his words, which suited me very well. So they did an ECG and sure enough I had a prolonged T wave, or something, I don't know – something to do with the repolarisation of the heart, whatever that is. But nobody has ever done a follow-up ECG to find out whether there is still any damage, and I agree there's not much point, because even if they found that there was some residual damage, what would they do about it? Frankly it doesn't bother me, because if I conk out tomorrow, I'll conk out tomorrow. I think another side-effect, although nobody was ever quite sure whether it was a side-effect of the drugs or whether it was an additional problem, was that I had epileptic fits around the mid-80s. I suppose the chances are it was probably caused by the drugs they gave me, but again it's difficult to say.

★ ★ ★

I was in hospital for maybe six years, on and off. The longest I was ever in at one stretch was 10 months. Some of the time my parents would come and collect me in the evenings, because we lived fairly close, seven, eight miles away, and we'd go back for a meal at home. Other times I'd stay in for two weeks at a time and never come out, it just depended how I was feeling. But yes, probably more in than out, and the periods I was in for varied quite a lot. I suppose the shortest would have been perhaps a month.

The voices got worse in hospital than they had been at university, which meant that at certain times when they were really bad I didn't want to go to sleep, and actually that persisted for years. You know how everybody has to go to sleep in psychiatric hospital, I mean you have to go to sleep you have no choice, you *must* go to sleep, so they dose you up with medication and so forth. One of the things they said, again I think I mentioned it in those sheets, was that if I didn't kill myself then I'd be dead by tonight one way or another. So I was terrified of going to sleep, so I didn't go to sleep. I mean I didn't really have any clear idea of what would happen if I did go to sleep, and I can't really say whether I thought that they would actually kill me while I was asleep, but it was unnerving anyway.

The voices continued pretty well all the time I was in and out of hospital, but they didn't change much in content. I know some people's voices actually get quite benign later on. Mine never got benign, they got a bit more tolerable. I think quite a lot of people can cope with the voices when they start, and what people tend to forget, quite apart from the content, is the length of time they go on. It's like a Japanese drip torture, where they drop water onto people's foreheads. I think most people could quite happily cope with it for five minutes, well not happily, but they could cope with that for five minutes say. In the same way I suspect that most people could cope with voices for five minutes, but it's really when you extend it that you begin to realise that it wears people down. And on that basis it doesn't in some ways really matter what they say, if it goes on for hours on end. I mean imagine if you carried a walkman around with you listening to Radio 4 all day; a better example – Talk Radio. Okay imagine that you had those in your ears, but it was invisible and you had to carry on a normal life with that – it would just drive you bananas.

It's the same with psychiatrists – they like to think that by sampling some of the drugs they know what the side-effects are. I was talking to one the other day, he was actually cooperating on one of these police training manuals, and he seemed quite proud that he'd actually taken some Largactil. Well I mean you can't do that, you have to stay on it for say two, three months to know what the side-effects are, because a lot of them are fairly long-term – the apathy and that sort of thing; weight gain, I suspect perhaps wasting of the muscles and goodness knows what. The idea that you can understand how patients feel by taking a few chlorpromazine tablets and having a really bad day the next day is ridiculous, and in some ways it's dangerous because it ignores everything but the physical side-effects. Sure the physical side-effects are bad, but the long-term side-effects, the social side-effects of the drugs, are as big a problem, and there is no way you can gauge those without taking the stuff for weeks on end.

★ ★ ★

In terms of recovery I was helped by a number of coincidences. Seeing the same consultant for 15 years – that's been very good. That's unique, as far as I'm aware. I've never come across anybody who's had the same consultant for that length of time, probably not for considerably less either. It happened because I saw him privately a couple of times; he was not the person I'd have seen normally because I wasn't in his catchment area, so it was a rather strange arrangement anyway, and there was no reason why it shouldn't continue. The other reason is that I just get on with him very well. Actually he's semi-retired now. He mainly deals with old people these days, so I'm on his patient list, but I think everybody else is over 60. And he was good – he knew when not to take any nonsense from me and when to give me a certain amount of latitude, which obviously helps. Another thing is that he was willing to discuss the drugs, and although he didn't quite recommend me to go and buy a copy of the BNF [British National Formulary], he had no objection to my finding out about them. I think perhaps he realised, which some of the nurses didn't, that here was a bloody awkward customer and nothing was going to happen except by my agreeing to it.

Being strong-willed I think has helped. Trusting my judgement in, say, rejecting advice from nurses who were no use, and discriminating between people who were going to help and people who weren't going to help me. I suppose you could extrapolate and say, well, maybe people who are bloody minded as children are more likely to recover. In a way that's what it boils down to. If they are strong-willed and stubborn, maybe it will make things awkward, but on the other hand maybe it's a strength as well. Maybe somebody who is more easily led is less likely to recover – maybe.

Another factor: having intelligent parents and a place to retire at home; those have helped. I mean some parents very naturally have inbuilt expectations of what their children are going to do. So for example my father was a doctor. He might have always assumed that I'd go into medicine. He didn't. But I think it's very damaging for somebody who's got any kind of mental illness to have expectations put on them by somebody else. So certainly that was a major factor – the fact that my parents didn't assume that I was going to do any particular thing, and they were quite happy for me to recover slowly, if you like, and there was no pressure for me to have a career of a set type and a set pattern. I certainly know of other people who've had schizophrenia who have not been quite so lucky; it's almost been accepted that they were going to do this or do that and – of course – great disappointment. Partly, obviously, guilt on the part of the person who's ill because they might not fulfil those expectations – and I suppose guilt on the part of the parents as well – who knows.

I took myself off medication eventually. My consultant was aghast, even though the doses had been dropping continuously. There's no way he would have done it. I don't think many psychiatrists are going to take somebody off medication for schizophrenia, because of course there is really no mechanism for giving somebody a clean bill of health, so it's a professional risk for a psychiatrist to do that. He risks being criticised by his peers even if it works – even if the patient's fine. So it's almost inevitable that if you come off medication you've done it yourself.

Possibly I gradually realised that I was capable of doing more and therefore the medication became less relevant. It took a long time, reducing the dose very, very slowly. My psychiatrist was very good. His first question was always, 'What medication are you taking?' when I went to outpatients. He didn't say: 'What should you be taking?', although he might say: 'Well, that's a bit surprising', or 'Maybe you should take some of this' or whatever, but he never assumed he knew what I was taking, even though he was prescribing it (well my GP was prescribing it, of course, but the consultant was telling my GP what to prescribe). So he never assumed I was doing what he said – which is very sensible of him because sometimes I wasn't. And I would always be totally honest with him about what I was taking. That obviously was partly because I had known him long enough that I could be honest with him. Of course gradually he came to realise that it was quite good that I wasn't taking as much as he was prescribing – in fact he did say once that he rather wished he'd started taking me off it earlier. I came off it finally I suppose it would be in 1993. Arguably I could have started coming off it seven or eight years earlier. It took years – and I certainly wouldn't advocate doing it in less.

★ ★ ★

The thing that probably helped the most was starting this voluntary work that I'm doing now. It started in 1989 I think, when my father, who's now retired, got involved with the National Schizophrenia Fellowship, and he was on the committee of that. The lady in charge told him they'd got problems with one of their computers in the office, and could I go around and have a look at it. Well, it was obvious beyond any doubt that this was useful to them, and I think that was the first thing I did since I'd got ill that was of value to somebody else. Nothing that I did in hospital was of value to anybody else, and of course much of it, such as the traditional sort of OT, was clearly of no use to anybody, because what was produced was thrown away at the end of the day – you could see it in the bin – so that was a waste of time. But when I started working for this charity that clearly was useful, because if I hadn't gone in they would have had to fork out quite a bit of money to get somebody else to do what I did, and that to some extent restored my self-worth... particularly since when I went into hospital I was given the normal thing, which is, 'You may have to be on these drugs for the rest of your life', and my parents were told that their expectations would have to change, I might not be capable of getting a job, ever. So when I started working for this charity it was clearly not true what had been said.

I've never had any formal training, which is a help actually in what I do, because I think it's rather important if you are going explain to people about things that you've made all the mistakes yourself first, and people who have a really good formal grounding may not have made those mistakes. I don't know whether it's anything peculiar to the computer industry, but an amazing number of user support people that I've come across are so supercilious and condescending it's just not true. So it does help not to have had any formal training with computers, paradoxically. I picked up the knowledge just by buying computer magazines every month, using the machines that I'd bought over the years, and just helping people use them at their work.

There is quite a variety in the work, so in some cases people will ask me what machine they ought to buy, that's a favourite question, and then what software they ought to buy; or they may ask what machine they need to buy and it may not have occurred to them it's important what software they buy – things like that. Then if things go wrong they will ring me up and say, 'Something funny is happening with this, do you think it ought to be mended or can you fix it?', so a lot of it is diagnosing things over the phone. And sometimes people ring up and say, 'I'm writing this document, and suddenly all the tabs have disappeared over the right hand side of the page', so it's just a question of talking them through it and telling them what to do, what key buttons to press, and try at the same time to include some explanation of why they are doing it, so if it happens an hour down the line they will be able to correct themselves later. But that's basically what it is; to a certain extent it's mending problems if they can be mended by me, explaining why things happen, why they don't happen, what they can expect from it. The thing that really pleases me is when people ask me how they can computerise some particular thing that they've got. There's a case in point with another charity, something to do with ex-servicemen. They had a very strange mobility card index system and they wanted to computerise it, and it was rather gratifying to tell them that they shouldn't, at least partly because they suspected they shouldn't. They'd been given some money to buy a computer so they could computerise this, but it was simply uncomputerisable if you see what I mean. Computers have their limitations and that's the trouble. People tend to regard computers as their job, when they should be seeing them as tools to do their job. I think the same may be true of psychiatrists and their drugs – their job isn't actually to prescribe drugs; their job is to help patients get better.

What happened was as far as work went, I was doing that thing at the Advocacy Group and other charities got to know about me so I'd start getting calls from really weird charities with strange names, and it ended up with quite a lot of charities. The one nuisance was that I couldn't actually earn any money from them – mind you most of them wouldn't have had any money to pay me anyway – but because I was on benefit, actually I still get benefit, it's really very limiting. I can earn about £15 a week, but that's all, so it's not worth collecting. Some places it's more bother than it's worth to actually claim expenses.

The other thing I do now is go around the country doing conferences with the NSF [National Schizophrenia Fellowship], and spin-offs like being on the Patient and Carers' Liaison Group at the Royal College of Psychiatrists. I will talk at conferences if people want me to, but I also do the hardware and the PA system if there has to be one. We show videos and quite often I'll hire a video projector to throw it up on the wall and I'm afraid I'm the only person there who understands how they work, which is going to be a bit of a problem when I get a proper job, which I hope to later this year. I don't know who is going to do it, but somebody is going to have to learn very quickly.

★ ★ ★

I think I'm probably a lot more self-confident with meeting new people since I was ill than I was before. It may well make you more self-confident I think – bit difficult to prove that, obviously, but it does teach you a bit about human nature. It shows you what people are capable of, so there's less unknowns for me now as far as people are concerned. And it does show the value of people – or lack of value. Certainly I wouldn't have held this view before I got ill, but I do now consider that people's worth as people is one – it's the same in every case, whether managing director or cleaner.

People do build up walls around themselves, and some people when they've been ill find it extremely easy to see through those – I certainly do. So it means that I can have a lot more sympathy for people than I would have before; in some cases a lot less patience maybe, because I can see there's really no excuse for some people behaving the way they do. I think I'm willing to make considerable allowances for people, but if somebody isn't prepared to pull their weight and is just trying to get sympathy for no good reason at all then, well, I don't have any patience with that. So there are benefits – or certainly there can be benefits for some people – though obviously the price is extraordinarily high to pay for any benefits. But nevertheless one can identify benefits and I think one has to because you'd get thoroughly fed up if you didn't.

PART FOUR

An insider perspective

Really enthusiastic about antidepressants: Stephen Goodfellow

Stephen is a health service psychiatrist working at a teaching hospital. He asked me to come and meet him at his counselling rooms as, he said, 'No one will know you're not one of my patients'. The stresses of his job and an ongoing manic-depressive illness don't seem to have taken too much toll on him. He is probably in his mid-30s, very likeable, lively, energetic and efficient. Sitting me down, he launched directly into his family history.

There's a long line of mental illness in my family. My great grandmother drowned herself in Morecambe Bay over whether or not to have the pork pie before or after the boat trip round the bay – she was thwarted in her desire to eat the pork pie afterwards and threw herself overboard on the trip and drowned, full knowing she couldn't swim. My grandmother, her daughter, was as mad as a hatter by the sound of things; she used to leave the house by the coal hole in the pavement because she felt there were people watching the front door, although she got better in later life. And then my dad was as mad as a hatter as well, indeed still is to some extent, and my sister is and so am I. So it's a good, clear family tree and we all have a bipolar affective disorder, although my grandmother sounds as though she got quite paranoid at times and I'm not, indeed I'm probably over trusting. And that's *not* why I became a psychiatrist actually, at least not overtly, because I didn't know I was going to have these kinds of problems myself until after I'd made that decision. So it wasn't any particular desire to obtain any degree of self-understanding.

I run a robustly biological view of bipolar affective disorder, which seems to suit me very nicely thank you. I don't necessarily apply it to my patients, but it's what I apply to myself. I respond exquisitely well to pharmacological treatment, thank goodness, and am well I guess 95 per cent of the time, although I run a sort of chronic mild hypomania, which is what we laughingly call my personality, but that's the way I am. And I get either higher or lower than that, more often lower which is a curious thing, you would think it would be higher being half way there already. And my sister tends to go lower as well.

★ ★ ★

My dad's a teacher, well he's retired now. He seems to have been much worse when he was younger; things got a lot better after he was about 50, but he had a chequered past with assorted problems. He seems to have been in jail in a wide variety of places, and had over 40 different jobs in about 10 years. It's very entertaining to hear him, but it doesn't bode terribly well does it? He was in the Merchant Navy, hence getting jailed all over the shop, but half the time I think he was jailed for just plain devilment or political things, rather than on the basis of any particular mental illness.

My parents had me ludicrously late in life, so that was all before I was born, it didn't affect my home life particularly. My dad was a bit erratic I think when I was a nipper because at times he was overly jolly and a bit free and easy with money and other times he was a bit miserable and difficult to live with, but probably not to any marked extent. He certainly didn't go around whacking any of us or anything like that. My mother's fairly level-headed and they are quite old now. And my grandmother had my dad when she was quite old, so she was always creakingly ancient, as long as I ever knew her, and more or less on an even keel, so there are only these apocryphal tales about quite how crazy she had been when she was younger, she never appeared to be so when I knew her.

I was the white sheep of the family in that I got a good set of A-levels and went on to university, although I was rather strange at school, but I think it's probably just native strangeness rather than anything else. I went to one of those hoity-toity places that gives you a good set of A-levels, but a terrible set of values, unfortunately, and my parents were very keen that I didn't acquire these snobbish values, which is fine, and I admire them for it, but it meant I spent most of my time at school bucking the system, permanently on the verge of being slung out, people thinking I was entirely outrageous and so forth. I wrote a scurrilous article once about somebody who was important in the school and whose parents mattered because they had money, and they were absolutely outraged and wanted whoever had done this ejected. But luckily nobody blew the gaff that it was me, in spite of the fact that it was widely known.

★ ★ ★

The school were very keen that everybody went to Oxford and Cambridge and so out of devilment I decided I wanted to go to London. I trained in a relatively unremarkable London teaching hospital and did okay, got honours in medicine curiously because I'd failed the medicine firm. I failed to answer this question on TB adequately and I had to resit it, and like a fool I read up what I failed on and then resat it, and of course something else came up, and I passed, it all went well. When it came to finals, what was the medical case but TB and I knew everything about it because I'd learned it twice, so I was able to give them reams of stuff about granuloma formation and ethambutol side effects and Mantoux tests, so I was up on the written stuff. Then my long case was on sarcoma of the femur. You can do a piece of surgery to try and chop it out, called a hinquarter amputation, which is a hideous thing; a fair number of patients die on the table and the others don't live any longer anyway, so no-one does it anymore. I was interviewed by the examiner, who said, 'Well is there any surgery you could do for this woman?' because I'd been talking at some length about her and how her husband was taking it badly, typical psychiatrist even then you see, more interested in how the relatives took it. I said, 'Well you could do a hindquarter amputation'. And he said, 'Would you let your mother have a hindquarter amputation?' and I said, 'Oh no, she's quite elderly', I said, 'I think it would kill her, besides there's nothing wrong with her; what an outrageous suggestion'. Luckily they took it the right way, not that I was being obtuse, and I must have tipped into the honours viva bracket there.

In London, you go up for oral examinations if you're meant to be outstanding in some field or other and they see whether you really are or you just got lucky. And I didn't give a toss because I knew I'd passed the finals, I was light of heart and fleet of foot. I tripped in merrily to this examination hall, and so that nobody knows who you are in case your dad's professor of something, not that mine is, you are all done by numbers. They said 'Candidate number 3792' or whatever and I said 'Yes', and they said, 'Now what can you tell us about Hodgkin's lymphoma?', and I said, 'That's my name actually', and they said 'What, Hodkgin?' And I said, 'No, no, lymphoma, ha ha', and

roared with laughter and luckily they did as well and I think that was sufficiently entertaining because I got the honours. I was so glad I did, because
throughout house jobs I applied to the most prestigious medical SHO [senior
house officer] posts, and they had to interview me, but as soon as I arrived it
was obvious I could just about name the organs, so I never got the job, but it
meant I took successive days off house jobs and they had to let me off and pay
me. I got about 14 days off in six months on the strength of going for these
extremely prestigious jobs.

★ ★ ★

I first got depressed when I was at medical school, quite briefly, and it got
better without any particular treatment although it was quite alarming at the
time. Looking back, I had a marvellous constellation of symptoms, I could
have written myself up. I have a copy of some correspondence that I sent to my
oldest and closest friend, and it was an absolutely classic sort of letter from
somebody who is depressed. It lasted about a month and a half. The registry at
my medical school, in view of my dismal family history, sent me off to see one
of the psychiatrists where I trained. He was fairly guarded and wanted to keep
an eye on me and indeed I duly got better. Then house jobs, which is when you
would expect anything to get set off – ghastly, a third of house officers are
clinically depressed, you work about 110 hours a week as a matter of routine,
and the most I worked was 196 hours in one week. I can remember how awful
I felt physically, but mentally I was fine, absolutely fine.

I was fine for a year after that, so you can't say that as soon as the stress is
off you fall all over the shop. Then the year after that I got problems; I was
working as a psychiatrist at another teaching hospital, and I was in a fairly
grim state, feeling very like boo-hooing in the clinics and indeed actually
boo-hooing in the clinics at one point. My decision-making powers were not
what they could be, so my judgement was a bit off as well, I suspect. The
person I was working for at the time noticed this and sent me home, which
was a wise move, and I got better again but it took rather longer this time,
about two months after that. I was only off work about a week, then went
back looking fairly grim and doing not as much as I did before, which was
silly really because if they'd had their wits about them they would have (a)
made sure that I got treated properly, and (b) not let me go back to work. It's
like having somebody walking around with an infectious illness isn't it, they

infect everybody else and don't do their job properly. You get rubbish health care if you're a doctor, particularly if you have psychiatric problems.

Then I moved here and did okay for about 18 months, and then blow me down, but my mood began to gently rise. And this was in the end spotted by the crisis intervention team across the road, but by that stage I was kind of ebullient, even more talkative than normal, eating two pizzas at midnight and a bit disinhibited and so forth, and things didn't seem quite right. And like sensible people, they immediately told my senior registrar of the moment who, like a sensible person, immediately told the hospital hierarchy, who officially said, 'You don't seem to be really quite all right'. And I'm very glad they did, because otherwise you can embarrass yourself tremendously, spend your way through a whole lot of money and make some terribly poor decisions. So they laid me off for a week and told me I couldn't come in even if I felt terrific, because that was the nature of the problem, and to see how I felt at the end of the week. By that time I was actually beginning to get better again, so I went down to the psychiatric crisis team and said somebody working there had grassed me up to my senior registrar; they were all quaking in their boots and nobody wanted to say who it was, but I said, 'Whoever it was I'm very grateful'.

★ ★ ★

I did all right after that for a spell, and then I was doing child psych, which isn't particularly challenging, or wasn't where I was doing it, and I began to get depressed, worst time ever in my life. I got worse and worse over the course of about three months of a six-month job and I developed the wooden facies of depression and the failure of sense of humour. No problems sleeping, but marked problems with appetite; at the time I was taking some antibiotics for something or other, and I developed the idea, God knows why now, in retrospect, that I had a *globus hystericus* lump in my throat so it was hard for me to swallow, and that was what was putting me off eating. After about three days I was ketotic, so that's when the penny began to drop, but I'd been in a poor old state for some time. Now bear in mind that at the time I was working for two consultant psychiatrists, and five psychiatric social workers and a clinical psychologist were working in the department with me, and none of them noticed. Startling isn't it? Worrying really. I could have been stringing myself up before they'd have noticed, then they'd have noticed I was strung up. They didn't say anything *except* for the head social worker. Because they'd noticed I'd become rather humourless and grim and cynical, this chap drew me aside and explained that he'd been deputised to come along by his colleagues to say that they were very worried about me because I looked like the kind of chap who didn't like his patients and I'd better improve my attitude. It's a great story isn't it, except that it's, like, not funny – it's true. So that was the helpful, caring sharing response I got from child psychiatry where I worked.

I was a little less than happy about that and just felt fairly wooden faced about it. I can remember distinctly having less spontaneous conversation and not smiling, I mean I could do if I thought about it, but it didn't occur to me to smile. I think my driving was probably not what it could be. I was not particularly tearful, kind of a bit slowed down, marked poverty of ideas and slightly decreased rate of thoughts. And the things I was supposed to be doing work-wise all became a huge effort, so it was only with the utmost effort that I managed to do anything. The people who did notice were my peers here, my friends indeed, and they all thought that things didn't seem to be quite right, but they didn't say anything. It just shows you see, even your closest friends don't tell you these things when they need to, and bear in mind these people are all psychiatrists, so if anybody would tell you, you would hope that they would. In the end they said that I didn't seem to be quite right really and had I talked to my other half about it? And because she's with me all the time, I was no different really any one day than the day before, so I gradually subsided down into a terrible state and actually she was probably in a similarly grim state at the same time because these things are just infectious really, not in a contagious sense, but it's very depressing being with somebody who is depressed. I developed a sort of psychomotor retardation in the end, where you slow down in both thought and motion. I was probably admittable actually.

I can remember one weekend, we were both walking up the road to the nearest urban centre to where we lived. I always get a vivid mental image of Lincolnshire in late autumn where my grandmother used to live when I'm depressed, because it's a combination of Somme-esque seas of mud, old wooden sticks with no leaves on them, a bitterly cold wind and everything being rather muddy and damp and unpleasant, with an overcast sky – sort of hell on earth for me. Anyway that's how I felt, and we were both walking up the road to our nearest urban centre, feeling like that and I said 'If I feel like this in a week's time, then I shall start taking antidepressants'. I wasn't entirely serious when I said it, but it wasn't a joke, because I hadn't got any sense of humour by then. We continued to trudge up the hill and we looked like crap really and trudged back again, and the next week I did.

★ ★ ★

By and large you shouldn't treat yourself, particularly not with any psycho-active compounds and I can assure you that now I don't, but I did then. I took sertraline, that ever favourite SSRI, chosen because it has fairly minimal side-effects and is not likely to precipitate mania, whereas TCAs do, so rational prescribing all the way. I'm actually very good at my job, even when treating myself. So none of this namby-pamby building up the dose, I just thought, 'Right, start off with 150 mg, which is top whack dose', I thought, 'Can't carry on like this', I think I was probably getting just a hint suicidal actually. It produced mild nausea, but not too bad, live with that, and retarded orgasm, which is another side-effect patients never tell you spontaneously, you have to ask them, and failure of yawn and sneeze. And I duly got better, like clockwork. Like clockwork.

I can distinctly remember the first time I began to feel better. You don't get better all at once obviously, life's not like that. And equally, you don't get better really gradually; what you get is episodes of feeling all right in a general sea of crapness and then the episodes of alrightness spread until you get epi-sodes of crapness in a general sea of alrightness, so it's like an Escher picture, where one turns gradually into the other. I can remember walking out of the door of the hospital and down some steps to go to a child psych seminar and I jumped over a chain, simply out of that kind of *joie de vivre* thing that you do when you jump over a chain, it was an enjoyable sensation, I can remember it now, one of the strongest sensations. It lasted until I got upstairs to the child psych seminar, and was gone. Now I'd forgotten how it was to feel like that because it had been literally months and months since I'd felt anything like it at all. That brief moment of feeling all right, in comparison to the general sea of shitness that I had around me, seemed like quite an ecstatic sort of thing. Then over the course of the next few days I actually did get better. I generally felt the seas of crapness receding, leaving a general whatnot of alrightness. I actually took a holiday then.

★ ★ ★

I went off on holiday and I duly took with me the antidepressants, because you should take these things for about six months otherwise you are likely to relapse. But being a sensible sort of fellow and having a terrible family history and having had what was almost certainly mania earlier on, I took with me haloperidol as well, because we went on holiday to Thailand and I thought if I get mania in Thailand it's going to be the end basically. So there I was in Thailand, taking these SSRIs, which are not likely to precipitate mania, no more likely than just chance, and I did. And I did. Most unfortunate.

I began to sleep less well and become even more talkative than I normally was and just like before my appetite increased, it either vanishes or it trebles, kind of thing, depending on which way I'm going. And my other half can distinctly remember me tucking into my second bowl of buffalo curd and treacle, a well-known Thai delicacy, and being annoyed that the waiter wasn't bringing me my third sufficiently rapidly and proposing standing him up to a fight over the matter. I'm not normally that kind of person, and she thought, 'Yes, this is definitely not right'. She said, 'You ought to be taking these haloperidol tablets because you're not right', so I duly did, and developed a dystonic reaction in the middle of an elephant orphanage, very unfortunate. I can tell you that these things don't hurt, although they can be alarming, though if you know what's happening it's not even particularly alarming, just inconvenient, and socially embarrassing. I got a dystonic reaction which affected my feet so I seemed to be only able to walk on the sides of my feet, a bit socially naff. So I duly crunched up my procyclidine tablets and took a mixture of the two instead thereafter and I was quickly all right. It's a very good antimanic drug, haloperidol, it seems to have some fairly specific effect. So we got through the rest of the holiday without any bother, indeed it was great, enjoyed it tremendously and I was more or less better by the time I got back.

★ ★ ★

When I came back from Thailand I was working as a duty doctor at another hospital site, a pleasant, rural sort of place. It has a duty doctors' flat which is nice, with a telly and a kitchen and a bed, because it isn't that busy. So there I was and I thought I'd do the dishes, because everything just piles up in the sink, you know, no cups, huge festering mounds of dishes, so I thought, 'Sod it, I'll do the dishes'. So I went to the bottom drawer in the kitchen in order to get one of those scoury things, and I nearly pranged myself. In the bottom drawer of the kitchen was a syringe filled with a [drug] depot, with a needle on it, and I thought, 'Who the bloody hell put that there and why is it there', so I thought, 'better dispose of this'. I thought, 'Can't put it in the bin because they have plastic bags and the porter will prang himself', and I thought, 'Can't put it in the sharps bin because this is a flat, there ain't no sharps bin', and I thought 'Well I can't really wrap it in newspaper and put it in the bin like it's broken glass or something. Shall I try and bend the needle into a complicated formation? No, no'. So I thought, 'I'll put it in the sharps bin on the ward'. So I put it on top of the telly to do in the morning. In the morning I forgot, thought no more about it. Three days later – frantic phone call from occupational health, what did I mean by endangering the lives of women and children by leaving a needle around in the duty doctors' flat? I said, 'Terribly sorry I forgot', and I explained. Anyway about three days after that I received a letter from occupational health saying they'd lost my occupational health questionnaire thing, which you fill in when you are employed in the health service, which I had duly filled in; they wanted me to fill out another. So I thought, 'This doesn't sound quite right to me. I think they're just having a snoop around here'. So I thought, 'Better be honest about this', so I filled the thing in, and I was rigidly honest. I admitted that I'm short sighted and dammit I can't read anything further down than the third line on the Snellen chart without my glasses on, that I have asthma, that I have atopic eczema, that I had ingrown toenails and so on, every little jot and tittle, I admitted to it all. And of course I was equally honest in admitting all the sort of problems that I'd had psychiatrically, which weren't that much. I mean, I'd had about three weeks off work in the course of my working life, it's not the end of the world.

★ ★ ★

I was summoned up to the occupational health clinic where they were taking my blood pressure and seeing whether it was true that I could read the third line on the Snellen chart without my glasses on. And the consultant fished me in, and she went through all the asthma and eczema sort of nonsense. And then she got down to the meat of the matter. 'Well', she said, 'It's this needle and syringe business'. I said, 'I don't know why you are worrying about it, it's a syringe full of oily stuff in a psychiatric hospital, it's going to be a depot, isn't it?' and she said, 'Well, yes. But all these psychiatric problems that you've had, don't you think that you ought to see somebody?' So I said, 'Well possibly'. She's right – I probably should. So she reckoned I should see Dr so-and-so, who's a professor at some other establishment, and I said, 'Well I don't want to go and see him; I might want to work there; I don't want him to be interviewing me and thinking, "He looks familiar, oh yes, I see him in outpatients"'. So I said, 'No, I'll see Professor somebody else who works here, if you like', and reluctantly went to see this man.

Now this professor was very good and thoroughly honest with me because he told me occupational health had tested the syringe for all sorts of opiates and stuff. I thought, 'Gosh'. I was amazed. I mean if I was going to go around shooting myself with heroin I don't think I would leave the syringe on top of the telly in the duty doctors' flat, it would be a bit inept of me wouldn't it? So I said, 'Why weren't they a bit more honest with me?' It would have been better if they'd just said, 'Now look here, we've tested this for opiates, because we want to know whether or not you are shooting heroin. Are you?' Rather than just sending me off to somebody else and simply regarding me with narrow-eyed suspicion, now we know why he's quite as strange as he is. So I went back to the occupational health person and I said, 'Now look here', I said, 'I understand that you've been busy testing the syringe for drugs; you could perhaps have told me, let's be frank and open about this. And besides', I said, 'any oily compound in a syringe in a psychiatric hospital is going to be a depot isn't it', I said, 'And it was a depot wasn't it?' And she said 'Oh yes it was, but we assumed that you'd been giving yourself a depot to treat your mental illness'. 'This is crazy', I said, 'Why would I be giving myself a depot, am I afraid I won't turn up at my own outpatients clinic or something? I won't attend my own appointments? It's crackers. I told the person on the sheet that I filled in that when I got mania I took haloperidol tablets, so why would I be giving myself a depot and most particularly why would I leave it on top of the telly thereafter if I was supposedly all right on it? This is absolutely mad'. Anyway, ha, ha, occupational health are well aware of what's going on.

★ ★ ★

So the story continues, this is good this: the chest X-ray. It leaves the psychiatric bit aside, but it's still funny, so I'll tell you it anyway. Among other things they said, 'Have you had a BCG?' And I said 'No', because I hadn't. When I went to medical school they gave me one of those skin test things to see whether I'd had TB and it came up positive, so presumably I'd been exposed to TB at some point in the past and got it and got better, the way most people do, and I felt fine, no cough or losing weight or stuff like that. I went all the way through medical school on the strength of this, without anybody worrying about it, but now that occy health got their hands on me they said, 'We want to give you another one of those', and I said, 'Well I don't want that, you see, because the last time I had one I had atopic eczema', I said, 'and it will probably come positive 'cos it did before, so there's no point in doing it'. So they said, 'Well in that case we'll give you a chest X-ray'. I said 'I don't want you to give me a chest X-ray, I feel perfectly well', I said, 'You may as well fish in someone off the street and give them a chest X-ray, I thought we gave up mass chest X-rays at the beginning of the 1950s on the grounds that it caused more breast cancer than it caught TB'. This has raged on, this issue, and now whether or not I continue to be employed here to some extent rides upon whether or not the occupational health department are prepared to let me get away without having a chest X-ray. Between you and me if it comes to me being fired I'll have a bloody chest X-ray, but as a matter of principle I can't quite see why they are X-raying me, other than that they've singled me out for these completely unconnected reasons, and I also suspect that the consultant who wants to X-ray me, because she looks at me in a funny way, I don't think I'm being paranoid here, I think she thinks that I'm crackers you see, not unreasonably, and I think she thinks that a chest X-ray would reveal something which I wouldn't want to reveal, such as Wormwood Scrubs '77 and '78 tattooed on my chest or that I've inserted razor blades under my skin or all my ribs have been broken in the past or I've got two hearts or something. I think she also thinks that I'm the kind of chap, because I'm so erratic and barking mad, that I might go around brewing up consumption just for a jape, you know, just to piss her off. Nothing could be further from the truth, I intend to stay well sort of thing.

But it's a point of principle now. Actually I would be even more up in arms if I were female, because you've got a one in 12 chance of getting breast cancer so you don't want some git toasting you with radiation on the off-chance. The chief radiation exposure for members of the general public is unnecessary medical X-rays, its not Sellafield or the ozone layer or Concorde or irradiated peas in the supermarket, or anything like that, it's actually X-rays by doctors. So I don't see why I should get toasted up on a whim, as though it's some kind of treatment giving you a chest X-ray, but I've tried to be reasonable about it. So watch this space, we'll see what happens.

★ ★ ★

When I was at medical school I wanted to be a cardiologist, because it all seemed quite interesting, but in the end I realised that one muscle, four chambers, four valves, two veins, three arteries, it's hardly a specialty really, is it? There is not much to it. Psychiatry was interesting because by and large the patients were more interesting than their illnesses. Can you imagine being an orthopaedic surgeon for the rest of your life, or in ENT, coughs and sore throats? It would be a bit brain numbing, wouldn't it? I suppose in psychiatry essentially you make your own judgement about what's wrong with the patient at an empirical and human level without following any particular protocol. If you are an endocrinologist and you think somebody might have Addison's disease you do X, Y and Z tests, which gives you A, B and C; depending on these the patient has or hasn't got Addison's, then you give them treatment along P, Q and R lines and if that doesn't work you try something else. So it's protocols you see, it's in a book, so if you read the technicalities of how to do it *you* could do it. Whereas psychiatry is not quite like that, and the only specialty I can think of which is similar is pathology, where you just get your slide and you look at it and you make a judgement about whether it's malignant or not. It's completely the reverse from the general public perception of pathology which is that somewhere there's a machine you put the slide in and it says 'Bing! malignant', or 'Bing! benign'. It's not like that at all, it's just a judgement made by some person, and another pathologist may make a different judgement. So psychiatry's the same, it's not as woolly as it sounds, and I quite like that. And I quite like the interpersonal aspect of it.

★ ★ ★

I went into psychiatry straight out of house jobs, then I did assorted little psychiatry jobs, then I went to another teaching hospital, then after that I came here, where it's been excellent, absolutely great. Had a marvellous time, met all sorts of interesting people and learned a great deal of useful things, very enjoyable and encouraging. And in the course of my duties I've dealt with a fair number of sick healthcare professionals, all of whom have received absolutely rubbish treatment everywhere else, because they either don't get seen at all or they are treated as special patients, and that's disastrous. Disastrous. It's like if you're a doctor and you have an operation in your own hospital, it *will* go wrong because the surgeon will be more nervous and he'll have shaky hands for a start, then the nurses do things different to what they normally do in the hope that they will be doing you a favour. Now they may be doing you a favour or they may not be doing you a favour, probably not is the answer, but they don't know what's going to happen. As soon as anything is done outside the normal treatment pattern, you're on completely uncharted territory. It happens all the time.

And if you're a doctor, particularly if you have a psychiatric illness, nobody is sure whether to treat you as if you're a doctor or a patient, so they're not sure whether to call you doctor so and so or not. The doctor treating you is nervous because you probably outrank him or her, and if you're a psychiatrist you might disagree with the treatment. And the nurses are really not sure what to do, are you going to be telling them what to do or are they going to be advising you what to do? So they are completely at sea, completely at sea. So most of the treatments we've got in psychiatry are all worked out in a doctor–patient setting and they don't work in a doctor–doctor setting at all. Half the trouble is if I went raving mad right now, they would have to admit me to this hospital, wouldn't they, and I'd know all the people looking after me, and it's very difficult to be looked after by people you know. And most doctors don't live in the catchment area of the places where they work, so they'd actually be admitted somewhere else, then they get the problem of being a celebrity patient, so they get a room on their own so nobody watches them as they hang themselves. Or they get sent to a private hospital, that hap-pens a lot, and then they get rubbish treatment very expensively, at the taxpayer's expense. We admitted somebody who'd spent something like 13 weeks in the Charter Nightingale on a section, not getting better at all. They were off their section within about 10 days of arrival and they were out within eight weeks and they're fine, working as a nurse in North London again without any bother, so you get rubbish treatment, rubbish.

We don't deal with doctors with drug problems, because the drugs units treat them independently, and there are endless droves of drug addict doctors, that's just par for the course. The rate of drug abuse is *dramatically* higher among doctors than it is, say, among lawyers, a similar professional group in many ways, but it's hardly surprising really, because you've got access to drugs of abuse, haven't you? Now the mental illness rate as such is a bit higher in junior doctors but approaches normal as soon as you get above about SHO, registrar level, so presumably people drop out or get better or don't rise through the grades possibly. Interesting behaviour, like they keep on working no matter how ill they get, so lots of people we admitted, like detained under the Mental Health Act, who were as mad as a bag of rats, were working the day before. Anorectic people who were in such a frail state that they were having trouble pushing the brake pedal in their car, who were still working. People who were *absolutely* crazy, people who'd got the DTs, they were popping Heminevrin and still working, so they'd *work* up to the mark these people. Indeed I had the same history myself, even though you're not well, you keep on working, very duty driven. What else do they do that's rather peculiar? Tend to self-treat, badly.

They tend not to self-treat very well because they can't prescribe; the doctors don't self-treat very well either. The ones who aren't psychiatrists get the doses wrong and so forth. And there's more to it than just giving tablets, as I'm sure you're aware. A lot of them are not nearly as sorted as you might think. One patient stands out in my mind distinctly. Singularly attractive, middle ranking, seniorish junior doctor. Actually I know somebody who works with her, and they're always very envious of her because they say she's strikingly attractive, she's got a rather thrusting forward sort of career, a going places sort of person and 'Oh she's so bloody perfect'. She's not so bloody perfect, because in fact she has a rip-roaring bulimia nervosa, is a complete nervous wreck and repeatedly deliberately self-harms – and they bleed themselves in an interesting way. Instead of cutting themselves they shove needles in their arm and extract 50 ml of blood, and this woman would then leave it in a glass on the bathroom shelf where she was living, disturbed behaviour to say the very least, but she still looked great at work and did her job very well thank you. So some of these people are spectacularly messed-up and still working, it doesn't stop them.

★ ★ ★

There is more to this game than meets the eye. What the cutters characteristically describe is rising feelings of tension and unhappiness which are relieved when they cut themselves, particularly when they see the blood. Cathartic sort of experience. They're the people who cut themselves like that, whereas people with borderline personality disorders cut themselves more roughly and crudely, because they feel unreal and they cut themselves because it hurts and then they know that they're real. It's very common. Deliberate self-harm is the commonest reason for admission to hospital for females of anything at all, 100,000 people every year; the second commonest reason for men after heart disease. It's very popular. I've never harmed myself but I've seen lots of people who have.

From my experience and also from seeing an awful lot of other professional people with mental illness, one thing that helps is not keeping secrets, not having to put a good face on it all the time. If people know that you get ill in this way, you're actually less likely to get ill because you're not going to have to pretend that you're not. So it notches down the stress a good few notches. And keeping secrets in other ways doesn't seem to help: I was struck that out of 35 patients that I was seeing at one point in the clinic, five of them were women who were gay and hadn't told the people they were working with or their family, but were nonetheless sure that they were and were unhappy with the situation. And they were also all, bar one, from this evangelical Christian-y background, which is good because it's a very supportive kind of community, but this was the one thing that you couldn't tell them sort of thing, so it was really eating them up and they were in a terrible state. And the one who had done all right was the one who in fact on paper would do worse, because rather than being a bit depressed or dysthymic she had a rip-roaring bipolar affective disorder; she did absolutely fine because everybody at work knew that she was gay and that she had a bipolar affective disorder. She said at first they all looked at her anxiously as if they were expecting her to go mad next week, but then she didn't, and she didn't have to go around pretending and she was also able to talk about the problems that she had in her emotional life, which she did from time to time, and get quite useful degrees of personal support from people with whom she worked, so the stress was downed considerably, no sort of inventing fictitious boyfriends or wide varieties of female friends, when it's actually the same person all the time, I mean if you're gay you'll know all about this, it's a difficult lifestyle to maintain. So the advice that I would give is that there's no point making any great big secret out of it because you'll probably make it worse.

The advice I used to give to my doctor patients was, at all times to lie to occupational health if at all possible, because they are completely untrustworthy. However, try to be open with your colleagues, but wait 'til you're in. And never sign your contract, because if you don't like the way it looks after the first three weeks in the job you can ask for it to be changed, but if you've signed it you've accepted it, that's just a general principle. That's about it really. I did a locum job at another hospital, a locum consultant job as it happens, and I'd had dealings with the occupational health department there in a professional capacity, and they said, 'Gosh you're in a worse state yourself than some of your patients', but they were quite happy for me to work there, it wasn't a problem. They said, 'If you worked here permanently we would want to have some kind of monitoring arrangement in place', but that's what I've got here, it's just sensible.

★ ★ ★

The professor I see is very good. The deal is that I ring him up, write to him or meet him in the corridor once every three months and say I'm fine and will go and see him if I think I'm not. The other part is that he is not prepared to have any dealings with me unless my other half knows about it and is able independently to say that she does or doesn't think that things are all right. She's quite happy with that, thinks it's a very sensible arrangement and indeed she periodically threatens to phone Professor so-and-so if I don't shut up. Charming, eh? In fact I'm very diligent and if she said, 'I don't think things are quite right', I would go along to Professor so-and-so anyway, I'm very good that way. So that's the arrangement to date. It's a good system really.

It's not a big secret. People round here know and if anybody were to ask me I don't think I would deny it, but equally I don't necessarily want to put an advert in the newspapers about it and I don't tell the patients because I don't think it's of any particular benefit really. You don't necessarily understand what it's like any better. I've always found people with depression more irritating since I've got depressed myself. It's *decreased* my empathy. What it has enabled me to do is to sound really enthusiastic in saying, 'Antidepressants are a really good treatment and they are not addictive and they are liable to make you better', and it has meant that I use sensible doses of haloperidol in treating mania because there's no evidence that giving more than about 10 to 20 mg is any better than anything else, and the mega doses that some people employ are of no great benefit.

Nobody else has ever given me any kind of drug-based treatment, which is irritating really because if they had done I would have been better in 10 days, wouldn't I? But people are rather chary about it, because they can always pretend and you could always pretend, if anybody were to enquire, that you've never been treated for any form of psychiatric illness, and believe me it makes a substantial difference. Think I can get health insurance, or sickness benefit? It's a nuisance, I'm cheesed off about things like the insurance, and occupational health. But there are worse things in this life that could happen to me. After I had my brief episode of mania which the crisis intervention team here spotted I kept reasonably quiet about it, but in the end I came to the conclusion that it wasn't of any particular benefit and we spend all our time telling patients that it's no big deal, so it seemed a bit duplicitous to go around pretending that it wasn't the case. It's not the biggest deal in the world, I mean if you're in China you're not going to be able to marry if you've got a manic depressive psychosis. Very draconian legislation: you'll also not be allowed to have children, if you get pregnant then they'll terminate your pregnancy whether you like it or not. So thank goodness I don't live in China.

★ ★ ★

It doesn't seem to affect my employability particularly. I think employers probably look at how much time you've spent off work and how well you do your job. I do my job quite well actually, at least nobody is complaining about it particularly, and I don't have much time off work, certainly no more than three, probably more like two weeks off in 10 years, and that's with every kind of sickness altogether. I had two days of bad back and one day I went blind, I got corneal oedema. The medical staffing department in the hospital where I went blind were saying, 'Do you think you can work until 6.00 this evening?' 'Well no really you see because I am blind, it will impair my ability to work, it's going to be tricky, I am blind.' 'Well, 4.00 perhaps?' 'No really, you don't understand. Imagine if you put Blu-tack over your eyes: I am blind, I cannot see. When I go to the canteen I'm going to have to get somebody to feed me because I can't see the plate'. So I don't take time off work for trivia really, it has to be major league. I suppose, being serious, I've been sent home twice, so when I get mania I'm not very insightful, I have to be told, but I know when I'm depressed. When it's pointed out to me I know I've got mania, people say, 'You've got mania'. 'Gosh you're right, I have.'

If push comes to shove I'd be quite happy to have ECT. I'd rather have ECT than have a tooth taken out, that's for sure. Safe as houses. Because if you have a tooth taken out, you know who gives the anaesthetic don't you? The dentist! He's had pretty minimal anaesthetic training, which is a basic danger, whereas if you have ECT you have a proper anaesthetist, it doesn't seem to do anybody any harm. I don't normally have a ludicrously gung-ho approach to being treated either, so there are lots of things I don't want to have done, but ECT would be very popular. For instance, if I got depressed all of a sudden and there was some crucial event which I had to get through, like if I had to be best man at a wedding or something like that, I would have no hesitation at all. It buggers your memory up a bit, but so does being depressed. So it's horses for courses really.

I seem to respond well to treatment so far. The natural history of such episodes is to become more frequent and more severe, unless you take things like lithium, which I don't, and you might say, 'Why don't you take lithium?' Well because the mild chronic hypomania which we laughingly call my personality might go, which I would regret. However, I've always told myself that if I have more than about two episodes of mania in any one year, I probably will. With this kind of particularly close monitoring service that I have, in that all my colleagues know and Professor whatnot knows and my other half is eagle-eyed, I think I probably wouldn't get very ill for very long before somebody said something, so it's probably not necessary. I have no reason to believe that I won't be treatment responsive indefinitely.

Postscript

As the manuscript for this book went into production I tried to contact all the people I had interviewed some years previously.

Jane was achieving some success as an artist, with several exhibitions to her credit and a studio space. Cheryl and Keith had both had recurrences of their difficulties, but were basically fine, successful in their chosen courses of art therapist and self-employed journalist. Julie was continuing to follow a busy two-track schedule as a community arts worker and touring performance artist.

Steph I was unable to contact directly, but heard that she was still with her husband and they'd had a baby. Diane had developed further difficulties with bullying at work and was eventually obliged to leave.

Paul and Adrian had disappeared without trace. Graeme had built a successful career as a freelance software consultant doing contracting work.

Stephen's career was flourishing; his predisposition to hypomania now controlled on lithium following a repeat cycle of mania and depression.

Lesley had died after falling down a stairwell just a year after I met her.

The professional view

Working on all the wonderful, complicated and messy stories in this book raised a huge question mark for me over the notion of 'recovery' as applied to mental health crises. What does it mean to recover? Recover from what? From a clinical viewpoint, the concept of 'recovered' implies illness and cure, while recovery from mental distress isn't like that – it is more of a process of psychological development and, as such, highly subjective. I doubted it could ever be defined objectively from the outside.

In order to get more clarity on these points I decided to canvas views from two ex-service-user consultants working in the field of mental health: Alison Faulkner and Jan Wallcraft. They in turn recommended me to Piers Allott and Philip Thomas. The final contributor to this chapter, Mick Carpenter, I had been in contact with earlier when he kindly commented on the draft proposal for this book.

I asked them all about their views on recovery: what it meant and what might help or hinder it. I also asked for their views on the state of the mental health services – past and present, and their vision for the future. I have edited their replies for inclusion here.

Strategies for living with distress: Alison Faulkner

Recovery of course is very variable, since everybody is very different. And of course it depends what you mean by recovery. I view it in terms of finding strategies for living with distress. We all experience distress in different ways and at different times. It may be that we get over-anxious about things, or we may have periods of depression – whatever. I think we don't acknowledge as a society that we all have mental health issues at some level. But everybody has mental distress – it's a fluctuating thing – and we need to find ways of managing that.

The Mental Health Foundation Strategies for Living (SFL) Project (Faulkner and Layzell 2003), in which I was involved, is about service users doing their own research on living with mental distress. The SFL Project asks people: what do you find most helpful in managing to live with or recover from mental distress? Research has to start with people who've had experiences of mental distress and the mental health services. The SFL Project shows that it's possible to do research that's emancipatory and empowering in its aims, its process and its outcomes. Research into the mental health services needs to be done properly with service users very much at the centre. Users need to give proper consent. And we need to ensure that service users themselves ask questions that they need answers to – research can otherwise miss key questions on any given topic.

The SFL Project doesn't require people to have been in hospital to be involved as user-researchers. It's quite a narrow view to exclude people on these grounds, though of course it depends what you want to look at. In my experience there's not a huge difference in terms of a person's experience of distress. In fact one of the major things I've learned over the last few years is the levels of distress that some people can hold outside of the services. However, there is a difference in the level of disempowerment. It's quite extraordinary how you can get treated in a mental hospital, unfortunately – and that's hugely disempowering.

The state of the mental health services

From my own experiences of having been in hospital I wouldn't at all recommend it as a therapeutic option. Added to which, acute care has gone downhill over the years, partly as a result of the shift in emphasis towards community care. Greater resources are being put into this, and at the same time attention has been taken away from the acute wards. This has meant that the acute wards have become more and more about dealing with people with severe problems, people who are on the sharp end of need and distress, who are at risk of harming themselves and other people, so these wards have become really difficult places to be – particularly the inner city acute wards. That's what the Sainsbury Centre report (1998) says, but there are loads of anecdotal stories as well.

Vision for the future

I'd like to see more partnership developments, such as the development of advance statements saying what should happen to you in a crisis. An advance statement is a kind of living will that states what you have found most helpful when you have had a serious crisis; for example, what kind of medication you find most helpful and who you want contacted, and so on. That's one way in which that kind of partnership can happen. It acknowledges that we are experts in our own mental health – we've done a lifelong study in it after all – and this can be complementary to the expertise that the professional brings to the situation.

There should be less emphasis on diagnosis. Diagnosis is totally unhelpful. Some people I know have had about six different diagnoses and how has that ever helped them? I don't see why you shouldn't talk about problems. I don't have a problem using the words depression, for example, or hearing voices. These words describe something, whereas schizophrenia does not describe anything. It's perfectly possible for mental health professionals to work without using diagnosis. Phil Thomas does it – and he has brilliant insights into reducing 'them and us' boundaries [see p.187].

People also need help with self-management in terms of working out what the triggers are for distress. This is something people can be helped to do for themselves in terms of taking a greater role in managing their own distress.

Lastly, we need to reduce stigma. There is still a huge amount of societal discrimination. Insurance, health schemes and jury service all exclude people with mental illness, and obviously people can't get jobs and so on. All of these things should be challenged.

Alison Faulkner is a mental health service user consultant, and former head of the Mental Health Foundation Strategies for Living Project.

Relying on our own resources: Jan Wallcraft

People's recovery could be enhanced if the mental health services were aware of users' views of recovery and their needs. We have to keep on remembering and keep on pointing out that recovery can't be defined by mental health workers or policy makers. It has to be defined by individuals themselves, along with the strategies they've found for themselves that help them make their lives work better. Complementary therapies and spirituality have been part of my journey, and talking about positive strategies such as these lifts people's spirits rather than endlessly criticising ECT and drugs. The vision that sustains me is that if I keep on doing what I'm doing – telling people that we can rely on our own resources – then sooner or later people will get that message and we'll start to do that individually and collectively. We will all become experts in our own physical and mental and emotional and spiritual health, and the doctors won't have any job.

Community care was on the whole positive in that people can now expect not to be spending long periods in hospital, and instead can expect (and get) a decent level of community services. And lots of good innovations have happened, especially in the voluntary sector. There's lots of very good voluntary sector services, so people now have somewhere to go and make friends, have meals, get access to complementary therapies and counselling, and are maybe helped to get some training.

Acute services seem to have got worse rather than better: there's lots of evidence for that. They're under pressure, the morale is low, they are staffed by agency nurses who don't really know the patients. A lot of people there are violent, on street drugs, and a high proportion of people in there are sectioned, so people in there are getting a very bad experience. If you go into an acute ward in a first crisis it's not going to be good for your mental health – it's a very poor quality environment: it's not good for anybody who's feeling vulnerable. And they haven't really moved away from the medical model to any significant extent, despite community care. People are still channelled into getting a diagnosis and pressured to take medication. It's a Catch 22 situation: if you don't get the label you don't get any treatment, and if you do get the label there are usually drugs attached to that. And you need the label to get the benefits, get the housing, get access to community care and some chance to get a bit of therapy. It's just no good really. You should be able to get help because you need it, not because you've got a diagnosis of schizophrenia or manic depression.

It's pretty rough on women who have patterns of self-harm and so on, who get labelled as borderline personality disorder. It's just used to rubbish their characters and not really provide them with a service. I know a lot of women with that kind of problem – self-harm, suicide attempts, eating distress – and nobody wants to know. They're desperately unhappy and desperately needy and they're just not getting a service, or they're getting a rubbish service. There are reasons why they're going through that – it's usually based on having a horribly abusive childhood and abusive relationships. But it's hard for them to get the in-depth therapy that they need. They need something really consistent over a long period, not to have it threatened or taken away from them.

Vision for the future

There are lots of things we can do for ourselves, but we also need more
resources that we don't currently have. In particular, it should be quicker and
easier for people to get the information they need all round. And we should
have information early in our lives about dealing with distress: that people can
get deeply distressed and there are things you can do about it.

We also need loads more for people who've had an abusive childhood.
That applies to more than half of people who've been in psychiatric care, and
it's probably higher – maybe up to 90 per cent – in secure hospitals. It's not
widely recognised, although the NSPCC have lots of information on childhood abuse. Many people are afraid to face it as they think they won't be able
to deal with it, but if you've had an abusive childhood you are going to have to
deal with it.

> Jan Wallcraft is a mental health service user consultant, who wrote her PhD
> thesis (2001) on recovery from mental breakdown. Jan is a Fellow for Experts
> by Experience at the National Institute for Mental Health in England
> (NIMHE), now part of the Care Services Improvement Partnership.

Experiential perspectives are vital: Mick Carpenter

Problems arose in the mental health services because no resources were put in
from the mid-1980s onwards. Policy was all about closing down facilities and
saving money. The emphasis has changed over recent years with the decision
to invest. This has got the pressure groups on side. But in the process, the
government moved away from the notion of rights (rights to life in the
community) to concern with risk: with scandal and worries about the
right-wing press. The focus has shifted to limiting risk from and to the
seriously mentally ill, and legislation on risk. Thus the 1999 review of the
Mental Health Act was called for on a rights basis, but has been used for other
things, principally compulsory treatment within the community and concerns
with dangerousness.

There are some good things. The National Services Framework lays down
good practice guidelines that include recommendations on increased user
involvement. It's a good idea to have national standards as it gives people
scope to develop. Another good thing about the National Services Framework
is that it admits the existence of health inequalities. In the mental health context this means that mental health problems are linked to social inequalities.
But there's not much evidence that mental health problems receive much

attention within this framework. Targets are all about reducing mortality – so the only criterion they tend to see in the mental health field is suicide. But at least there is scope for people to say that health inequalities need to be addressed.

The mental health services' history

Psychiatric beds reduced from 150,000 or so (including learning disability) in the 1950s down to about 50,000 in the 1980s. Not just numbers were affected in the scaling down of inpatient services but also throughput, i.e. beds were more intensively used, creating a revolving door situation. This had a particularly adverse effect on the younger generation of patients, such as Christopher Clunis[1], who were not so well known to the services.

Despite the changes, attempts to treat people still took place within a rigid, hierarchical framework. So while the old mental hospitals were not particularly therapeutic, new mental health facilities can often still have the same problems. The medical model makes the assumption that it's not the institution but the drug that makes the difference, and the new acute units still tend to be dominated by this.

Research in mental health services

Psychiatry is one of the most problematic fields of medicine. But the only evidence we have of problems is anecdotal, from service users, since critical research has not been conducted by the services themselves. This user voice still needs to be heard.

Experiential perspectives are vital. Users should have much more control over research and should experiment with user-led research. Carers should be brought into the picture as well, as they have a stake. I would strongly support having research accountable to users, but as an academic I would defend the notion of expertise as well; it's possible to construct a partnership. We should

1   The stabbing and killing of Jonathan Zito by former psychiatric patient Christopher Clunis in 1992 was widely regarded as the most notorious example of the failure of the then Government's policy of community care. An inquiry found the health and social authorities guilty of 'a catalogue of failure and missed opportunity', and the incident contributed to a review of mental health aftercare which led to the introduction of supervision registers.

recognise that users don't have all the answers any more than mental health professionals, though we're still a long way away from achieving balance.

Mick Carpenter is a Reader in Social Policy at the University of Warwick who has worked for many years in the fields of mental health and social care.

In recovery: Piers Allott

The actual word 'recovery' (in the sense of recovery from mental illness) didn't come into common usage until the early 1990s, and particularly following the publication of Bill Anthony's paper, 'Recovery from Mental Illness: The Guiding Vision of the Mental Health Services during the 1990s' in 1993. In the 1990s the amount of recovery information and the number of recovery stories that were written grew exponentially. Then the consumer movement in the US and in New Zealand in particular began to do things relating to recovery. The recovery movement as it is now is to do with raising the consciousness of people who experience mental disorder or distress, which came out of the civil rights movement in the 1960s and 1970s. In a sense people who experience mental distress have been the last group of disenfranchised people to come forward. Compared to the women's movement, black power, disability rights movement, people with mental distress haven't taken control in the same way – and that's now more recognised in the Disability Discrimination Act and its US equivalent.

All these things have lead to the development of recovery-orientated services worldwide. Somewhere in the region of one-third to a half of states in the US now have recovery as policy. It's primarily people who've used mental health services coming together, putting the information together and identifying what recovery is, as far as it's possible to do that. In the state of Ohio, for example, you will find that recovery is the policy of the state, and not only that, but they are currently in the process of implementing a recovery-orientated outcomes measurement system, because if you get recovery as policy then it's reasonable to ask: are we enabling people to recover? And if you ask that then you've got to have some means of trying to identify or measure it. New Zealand have produced recovery competencies for the mental health workforce, which sets a definition of what recovery concepts are and what is expected of the workforce.

In recovery

Probably people who are dealing with their recovery best would never consider themselves to be recovered – they would consider themselves to be 'in recovery'. There's a problem with the word 'recovered' in my view, in that the concept of recovered implies cure – it's over, finished – whereas what you are talking about is a developmental process. The definition of recovery isn't one that excludes the possibility of having further psychotic episodes or other experiences of mental distress. It's about managing the experience, getting on with life, and finding ways of dealing with crises that may occur. For example, taking medication is a management strategy rather than an indicator of recovery or otherwise.

There exists a stubborn notion that if you experience a psychosis then you will need services in order to recover, whereas the reality is that there are people who recover from serious psychosis without ever having come near services. Equally, there are people who recover from psychosis who've been into the services once and decided they would never go back, and who instead develop their own strategies for dealing with it outside. There's a book, written by a psychologist in Hamburg called Thomas Bock published in 1999 in German, I'm afraid, which is a piece of research on 34 people who recovered from psychosis outside the mental health system. Within psychiatry there's some notion that if you suffer from psychosis you must have treatment, whereas in fact that's not true. I've just completed a literature review (Allott, Loganathan and Fulford 2002) and we have included several quotes from Thomas Bock in that. It's one of my ambitions to get his book translated, and since I have now found a translator who has agreed to do it, the book may well be available in English within the next year or so.

Development of recovery-oriented services

I've been promoting the concept of recovery now for 11 years. Until recently I was seen as being a little outside of the norm by mental health professionals, service users and their family members. Then I began a research project in 2000, which was specifically geared to bringing the concept of recovery into a UK context; that's what our literature review is part of. I also trained with Mary-Ellen Copeland in Vermont in the USA as a mental health recovery educator, and I now deliver Wellness Recovery Action Planning (WRAP) workshops, and with colleagues have delivered two five-day WRAP and Recovery Educator (training for trainers) programmes.

My focus is to try to teach people who experience mental distress that it is possible to recover, to teach them how they can do that and how they can get what they need for their recovery – and that's the way we train mental health professionals. If people who experience mental distress come together and work with each other to recover from their experiences, then they have the power in their own hands. We had a recovery network in the West Midlands and there were professionals within that network, but those professionals recognised that recovery is something that people who experience mental distress do, whereas support is something that professionals do; and those who don't believe in recovery don't get involved. There's a parallel with cognitive behaviour therapy: it works for some people, and parts of it work for a lot of people, but it doesn't work for everybody. If professionals begin to recognise that there isn't a simple road to recovery, then they'll realise that you can't systematise it.

It's my belief that if we changed one thing in psychiatry today, we would lose 20 per cent of the population in secondary care mental health services. That is, if every psychiatrist who was making an assessment and giving a diagnosis of severe mental illness actually told people that recovery was possible, and gave them hope that they could recover, 20 per cent would go off and recover without psychiatry. We know from traditional longitudinal research that between 46 per cent and 68 per cent of people with severe mental illness recover, and we've known that since the early 1970s. The problem with psychiatry is that most of the research is short term and carried out on people who are experiencing severe psychological crises and in hospital at the time. If you look at any individual at the worst time in their life, that can't reflect who the person actually is. With longitudinal research you look at a person over the course of their life and you find that people do recover.

> Piers Allott is former Recovery Advisor to the Department of Health on mental health, and National Fellow for Recovery at the National Institute for Mental Health in England (NIMHE). He is based with NIMHE East Midlands.

Casting off the mantle of oppression: Philip Thomas

The single most important obstacle to recovery for many people who are in contact with mental health services is the medical model, which runs alongside the use of a strictly scientific approach in psychiatry. Although the two are not the same, the former is largely dependent on the latter. If you look at how most psychiatrists think, talk and act around a person with a diagnosis of schizophrenia, it is as if it's never going to be possible for the person to be free of that label. Even though you may show no signs of the condition, and you regard yourself as 'recovered', a psychiatrist will tend to think of you as someone who is vulnerable and liable to future relapses. It makes no difference what you might think yourself; your future possibilities are being defined for you in a very powerful way. For this reason, if mental health professionals and psychiatrists in particular, are to have any role in promoting mental health, they must abandon the medical model. This is the first step towards working in a way that helps people. Only if professionals do this will it open up the possibility that somebody can recover.

But there is more to it than that. There is a problem of definition. If we say someone has recovered, we have to ask what it is they have recovered from. The word recovery in this sense implies that someone has recovered from an illness. In other words, the expression takes us back to the medical model. Recovery may also mean regaining one's health after an illness, but many people who experience distress feel that their lives are changed for ever afterwards. For these reasons it may be better to think of recovery as reclaiming the right to understand your distress in your own way, rather than in a way given to you by professional expertise.

Recovery in this sense is a powerful idea. It suggests that recovery is an active process engaged in by mental health service users, either individually or collectively, to take control for themselves. The Brazilian educationalist Paolo Freire makes this point in his book *Pedagogy of the Oppressed*. His ideas are based in his experiences of working with the poor and dispossessed of São Paulo, but they are relevant to the political situation of mental health service users. He argues that liberty cannot be gifted by the oppressors to the oppressed. Oppressed people have to grasp freedom for themselves.

Casting off the mantle of oppression

Each person's approach to grasping liberty differs. Each and every recovery journey is unique. This is why recovery is so complex. It has to be defined individually by each person. I strongly disagree with the view that recovery means a life free of symptoms. I have dear friends who are survivors, and who continue to battle and cope with extremely distressing experiences, but despite this have a very rich quality of life. Their lives are a tightrope between 'If I do this I know my voices are going to torment me', and 'I have to do this because it's important to me'. There must be no overarching notion of what recovery means.

This brings us back to Paolo Freire's work. Freire points out that the most important way the oppressed can take control is through joint action, which means having networks of support in which it is safe to talk about common experiences of oppression. In this way individuals overcome the isolation that follows from being excluded. This is vitally important, in my view, for people who use mental health services. This is why the work of the Hearing Voices Network is so valuable. It provides safe spaces where people can share their experiences and discover the meaning of their experiences for themselves. Meaning and understanding are important in these processes of taking control, and are achieved by sharing stories. Individual stories must be told and retold, told and retold a dozen times over, if necessary. Each telling to a different person brings in a different perspective, and new meanings emerge from this.

Psychiatry without the medical model

There is nothing revolutionary in saying that diagnosis is of no value in psychiatry. Psychologists like Richard Bentall (1990) and Mary Boyle (1993) have been arguing this for many years. Both argue that the diagnosis of schizophrenia is unscientific.

For nearly 15 years before I finished working as a psychiatrist I never used diagnosis. I found it an obstruction. Of course under certain circumstance it has its uses. It may help you to access services or benefits. Some people want a diagnosis because they understand their experiences in medical terms. Under these circumstances I don't believe I have the right to take that away from someone. I might want to explore it gently with them, looking for the possibility to get them to question it for themselves, and to raise other possibilities, but I would never take it away from them. In this sense diagnosis becomes replaced by something else: a search for meaning. And although I disagree strongly with the use of diagnosis in psychiatry, I also disagree strongly with those (often academic nurses) who argue that doctors have no part to play in helping those who experience madness and distress. In Western culture physicians have always played a symbolic role in helping people at times of spiritual or emotional crisis. The best recent examples are R.D. Laing, and those influenced by him, particularly the late Loren Mosher. The work of both these figures shows that doctors, like other helping professionals, *can* play a part in helping people find meaning in madness, as can – of course – people who have made the journey through madness themselves. It seems to me that a range of personal qualities, life experiences and understandings of human nature are essential to this, as is described in detail by Loren Mosher in his book (Mosher and Burti 1994).

Reducing 'them and us' boundaries

Some years ago I wrote an editorial, 'On the nature of professional barriers', in the *Journal of Mental Health* (Thomas, 1995). In terms of clinical work it makes no difference which branch of medicine you are working in, to some extent you have to be a chameleon to be a doctor. You have to be all things to all people. For example, many people want and expect their doctors to be remote and detached. They want clear boundaries, and so I would play that role to some extent. But for many people that aura of superiority, detachment and difference can be crippling; it represents a further rejection of them as a human being – so anything that can be done to break that down is essential. This has to take place not only at the level of the individual person, but also at the level of service user and survivor networks. For this reason my view is that psychiatrists need to do much more to establish really close links with their local service user/survivor networks. This means contributing to their activities if they want you to. It also means being prepared to go and listen to them, and to be shouted or snarled at in order to start breaking down barriers. It is only possible to establish trusting relationships with people if they feel that you can tolerate their anger. This is essential if barriers are to be broken down between psychiatrists and service users.

The value of talking

I want to come back to the importance of talking. I am not referring here to talking treatments or therapies. They work for some, but in my mind are greatly overvalued and potentially as harmful and damaging as biomedical psychiatry and drugs. The type of talking I am referring to here is that of telling stories. I have already indicated that this is essential if people are to come to terms with distress and make sense out of it. It overcomes solitude, isolation and stigmatisation, and develops and builds sources of solidarity with other people. This notion of solidarity is terribly important, and here lies one of the great strengths of the user movement, because it helps to bring individuals together and overcomes the sense of oppression and loneliness that many people share. Psychotherapy and psychiatry both see emotional distress as something that's located in the being or body of an individual person. They both ignore the importance of spirituality and cultural and social contexts. It is our culture and our spiritual belief that bring meaning into our lives.

Madness and distress can only be understood if we listen to people's stories within their spiritual and cultural settings.

Philip Thomas is a Senior Research Fellow in the Centre for Citizenship and Community Mental Health, University of Bradford. He is also the Chair of Sharing Voices Bradford, a community development project working with the city's black and minority ethnic communities.

Conclusions and practical advice

Mental breakdown is universally a traumatic experience in that it represents the extreme of what we humans can deal with. Breakdown can be extremely frightening, extremely isolating and disorientating; it can be very protracted; it can even be fatal. It always requires the utmost kindness, patience and empathic understanding from carers if any intervention is to be effective.

Aside from these fundamentals, each person's experience of breakdown is utterly unique. For some, there may be an abrupt, catastrophic cut-off of normal psychological functioning. For others, there is an increasing inability to cope with work or studies, or function effectively in looking after themselves or others. For some, there is an obvious background of childhood trauma or abuse. For most, there may be a distinct trigger that precipitates a breakdown, such as a loss or bereavement. The very ordinary nature of such triggers is remarkable, in that it indicates that no one can be immune. Some people may be more vulnerable than others, but all are potentially vulnerable *in extremis.*

Recovery from a mental breakdown is likewise an intensely individual journey, as diverse as the people going through it. It follows that – as with breakdown – there can be no universal template for the process. Keith points this out on p.58:

> Unfortunately there are no easy answers, there are no formulae: if you do this or do that, take this tablet or follow this set of strategies, you'll be OK.

One of the few defining features of recovery is its developmental quality. The process tends to be incremental, and slow. Slowly, we come to understand what triggers our distress and act accordingly. We get to know our weak points as well as our strengths; where we are likely to get stressed, what helps to counteract this tendency, and what other things can help to overcome our difficulties. Developing a greater degree of self-awareness is thus an integral part of the process of regaining well-being. There may be times when we still need the props, like Steph opting to continue with her medication. Equally, coming to see what doesn't help is part of the process. Then we can avoid those things, or remove ourself from a situation that is likely to cause difficulties.

Supports to recovery

Aside from this, two major factors seem to act as decisive supports to recovery. They are first and foremost the decision to recover – and to take charge of the process so that our life moves in a positive direction. Second, but also of vital importance, are relationships with others that empower and support our recovery.

Deciding to get better and to take charge of our recovery seems to be the single most important indicator of success in emerging from a breakdown. Support from others – mental health workers, friends or relatives – is often crucial. Ultimately, however, every person's recovery has to be self-directed. Graeme (p.150) is particularly clear on this point:

> Being strong willed I think has helped. Trusting my judgement in, say, rejecting advice from nurses who were no use, and discriminating between people who were going to help and people who weren't going to help me. I suppose you could extrapolate and say, well, maybe people who are bloody minded as children are more likely to recover. In a way that's what it boils down to. If they are strong-willed and stubborn, maybe it will make things awkward, but on the other hand maybe it's a strength as well.

Everyone has their own distinctive way of taking charge, which can have many different strands. For Jane, this involved taking long walks and eating carbohydrates at each meal. For Julie, it started with enrolling for training as a drama therapist, and later involved challenging a therapist and a GP who treated her disrespectfully. For Keith, it involved withdrawing himself from a vicious circle of overdosing on medication and alternative therapies. Challenging the mental health system may even be a necessary part of the process of finding our own way.

Empowering relationships are also of critical importance in recovery. These relationships may be with family, friends or healthcare professionals – and they may be brief interactions as well as long-term supports. All of the people I spoke with mentioned the great value of being listened to in a genuine way in which they felt heard, respected, and accepted for who they were. Paul, for example, who had been frustrated by his previous interactions with mental health professionals, finally met a psychiatrist who he felt heard him:

A couple of weeks later I was seen by a forensic consultant psychiatrist called Dr Bushnell, a very good doctor. He made about three or four lengthy visits, and he came up with quite a long report for the tribunal, because I'd appealed against the section 2... I'm very thankful for seeing Dr Bushnell because he was the most perceptive and understanding doctor, the first doctor who I felt knew what he was talking about – who was listening to me and made an accurate diagnosis of what was wrong. (p.134)

Lesley has a similarly affirming experience with the therapist she went to for telephone counselling sessions:

Rational emotive therapy is not a regularly used technique in this country, it's very much American – a cousin in a way of cognitive behaviour therapy... The emphasis is on your faulty thought systems and not how you feel. But it did help, sort of. I don't think it was RET itself, but just the fact that for probably the first time in my life I stuck up for myself. It was really hard work because this man irritated me... Saying that, he was very, very tolerant... I was really hard work myself... but he stuck by me and no-one had ever really done that before. I really value that whole period. (p.122)

For the majority of people, relationships with mental health professionals of some sort are often key to recovery (Allott 2002).

Critical to taking charge of our lives is the development of increasing self-awareness. This means feeling our feelings, which can often be terribly painful. Jane's is the most extreme example, when she's describing her recovery from psychosis. The psychosis seems to have served a purpose in shielding her from painful feelings:

We had a great long discussion... and I got very upset. I felt utterly betrayed. Everything that had happened to me I'd made sense of. All the unkind things and the cruel things, the way my parents had literally dumped me, and all those humiliating experiences in hospital, I'd turned them around so they were useful... I'd made it as if there was some point to them. Suddenly I realised that people had actually done all these dreadful things to me, and I felt awful, absolutely awful. (p.29)

Feeling our feelings can also enable us to avoid the build-up of stresses that we know might trigger a setback. Maybe doing something to take our mind off the problem will help, and Keith is eloquent on this (see p.57). In the end, however, we can't avoid mental pain – and going through it may even help us to be a better person – or at least a more complete person. Diane talks about this in discussing the benefits of attending a Kubler-Ross workshop:

> Realising, for example... that it's not a sin to have bad feelings, that it's best
> to accept them... So whereas in the past I'd have been terrified of negative
> feelings and tried to push them away, now I try to make friends with my
> negative side and then I can function positively – I don't get paralysed. I
> allow myself to feel what I'm feeling. (p.103)

For most people, recovery is a process that entails learning to live with
fluctuating levels of mental distress, as we all do – diagnosed mental health
problems or not. Thus for Cheryl, Keith and Stephen, it's a case of living with
a degree of instability and devising coping strategies to minimise the risk and
severity of further disruption. Such approaches have been advocated in
reports of several user-led studies (for example, Read and Faulkner 2001).
They are hugely diverse, from complementary therapies and spirituality to
counselling, creativity and the arts, and developing support networks. I will
just touch on one or two rather than going into detail.

Working our way out

Getting back to work was a critical component of the recovery journey for
Keith and Graeme, and important for several of the other contributors, among
them Lesley and Cheryl, who both enrolled in re-training. This is Keith:

> I suppose the way I am slowly but surely coming out of my black hole is
> through work. I am very fortunate in that regard because I am sure if I hadn't
> got any work, or been unwilling to go for self-employment, I'd probably still
> be in a very bad state. (p.57)

In Graeme's view:

> The thing that probably helped [me] the most was starting this voluntary
> work that I'm doing now. (p.152)

Clearly, finding something better to do is part of getting out of the rut of
being a psychiatric patient. It might be immersing oneself in work, as with
Keith, or volunteering, as with Steph, but it can just as easily be involving
oneself in music or the arts, as with Julie:

> I think my music saved my life, I really do... I like the idea of moving forward
> into something more spiritual with voice that picks up on that idea of having
> sound in every cell of your body. It beats the shite out of Prozac, I'll tell you.
> (p.75)

Helping others in difficulty is also a wonderful way out of our own distress – and one chosen by many of the contributors here. I found it really inspiring that several chose to work in the mental health services in order to improve the lot of other service users!

Medication – or not

Medication can be an invaluable support in times of crisis. However, it may not work for everyone; not every medication will work in every situation, and all of them can have side-effects, which become increasingly likely with higher doses. If we are feeling worse after taking a medicine than we did before, it may be that we are on too high a dose, or that we need to switch to something more suitable, which might mean another medication or equally a non-drug approach.

Coming off medication, particularly long-term medication, needs to be approached with extreme caution. Jane and Keith describe in graphic detail the horrendous side-effects they experienced after rather rapid drug withdrawal. Graeme is more circumspect:

> Possibly I gradually realised that I was capable of doing more and therefore the medication became less relevant. It took a long time, reducing the dose very, very slowly. My psychiatrist was very good. His first question was always 'What medication are you taking?'... I came off it finally I suppose it would be in 1993. Arguably I could have started coming off it seven or eight years earlier. It took years – and I certainly wouldn't advocate doing it in less. (p.151)

Implications for mental health practice

Continuing deficiencies in mental health care, and particularly in the acute mental health services, have been widely acknowledged in reports by the Department of Health (2001), the National Institute for Mental Health in England (NIMHE) and the Sainsbury Centre, among others. But to read about the defects and abuses from the consumer perspective is nonetheless shocking – and mental health practice comes in for considerable criticism in these stories. Part of it is undoubtedly due to the fact that some of the testimonies date back 20–30 years or more. Part may well be because six of the contributors were recruited through a mental health activist organisation whose remit was to challenge existing policy and practice in the mental health system. Nevertheless, we cannot dismiss their criticisms on these grounds. On the contrary, they give a unique perspective on the services from the receiving end, and highlight the fact that there remain inadequacies that need to be addressed. In my view, these inadequacies are not confined to the mental health system, but reflect a lack of understanding of mental health issues within wider society that manifests as people shutting out their own problems and adopting oppressive attitudes to those with a mental illness diagnosis. Implicit in this are two key antidotes: we need to recognise that we all have mental distress at some level, and that the wise response to it is one of compassion.

Supporting recovery: what helps?

What else do we learn from these stories that is helpful? Well, just being there in a kindly way is a valuable antidote to the profound isolation that people can experience in times of deep distress. Authenticity – being real – is also really important. This means listening to people in distress and responding in a genuine way; not treating them as illnesses or cases. Third, working with people to support their recovery in finding out what strategies work for them. Don't assume that drugs or ECT will be the answer in a crisis: they may not be. (ECT causes persistent memory loss in at least one-third of people, according to recent evidence (UK ECT Review Group 2003), so should only be used as an absolute last resort, if at all, at the insistence of the client.) Always provide information so that the person can make an informed choice. And finally, for the long-term good, work on challenging oppressive attitudes in the wider society, rather than colluding or just putting up with them.

Supporting recovery: what helps?

- Being there
- Being real
- Listening well
- Working *with* clients
- Going out on a limb – if necessary
- Providing information
- Challenging oppressive attitudes
- Working on own issues

Being real

All of my contributors, without exception, found the support of mental health professionals valuable on at least some occasions and key to their recovery in several instances. But in almost all cases where professionals were obviously and genuinely helpful, it's where they were stepping out of their prescribed roles and relating to the person in distress on a reciprocal, human level – in other words, 'being real' with the person. There's the RET therapist being there in the middle of the night to answer Lesley's phone calls. There's the psychiatric nurse who kept an eye on Jane and became a friend.

There's the strong relationship between Steph and her key worker, Laurie:

> The most helpful incident in my whole psychiatric career was when I went for my assessment for Hoxton. I went to see this nurse and it was Laurie that I met. He was supposed to be doing a half-hour assessment on me. I was still there four and a half hours later, so was he. That's nearly four hours of his free time that he sat there talking to me. (p.92)

There's a good example of a professional literally stepping out of their role in Jane's story, where she talks about coming off tranquillisers with the help of her GP:

> I cut [the Mogadon] down, and within five weeks I was off it. It was quite hard, because each time I cut it down I had a couple of sleepless nights, but I was so determined to do it. I'd really got to the stage where I had no alternative left. When I went back to see him, his jaw dropped. He said, 'You haven't done it have you?' And I said, 'Yes'. Do you know, he did the nicest thing. He got up from behind the desk and he came out and he shook my hand. And he said, '*That's* amazing, *well done!*' And that made such a difference, I couldn't believe it. It really helped, that, because it was hell coming off those things. (p.30)

Julie's story shows another case in point. She has gone back to her therapist to lodge a complaint after she unilaterally terminated their body work sessions:

> I went back to see [this therapist] because I was bloody furious. I went through this real grief afterwards. I said, 'You're a bastard', I just felt I needed to tell her. And she really touched me because she said, 'I'm so pleased you came back. I feel I made a lot of mistakes with you and I'm very, very sorry. I was quite disarmed because I didn't expect her to come off her pedestal, I thought that was brave and I really took it to heart. I thought. 'Oh, she's only a human being, after all, it's just a bloody job'. So I shook her hand and went on my way. (p.66)

By contrast, where mental health professionals are distant, detached, plain nasty, or in other ways not relating on a genuine, human level, it can lead to a person on the receiving end feeling alienated, dismissed, ignored, angry or dependent. It's worth noting that being real does not always or necessarily mean being nice: it can mean confronting issues within a relationship. This is Diane, for example:

> This psychiatrist was very tough. He said to me, 'I know you need to phone us, that's fine, but we'll make a contract. If you phone me I will speak to you, but it will have to come out of the time I see you as I don't have that much time to spare.' So while in the past I knew they'd get irritated, but nobody would ever say anything, he brought it up front and it made sense to me – I felt as though I was being heard and seen. Of course I didn't like it – I felt humiliated – but I respected him for being honest with me. (p.102)

It's impossible to put a formula on 'being real'. It depends on the characters involved and the situation. But certainly the value of good listening – by which I mean respectful and kind attention – cannot be overemphasised.

Providing information as required, particularly about the side-effects of drugs, is also important. And continuity of a relationship is a great help. Graeme, for example, describes how seeing the same consultant for 15 years, and being treated respectfully by this doctor, was a key factor in his recovery.

> He was willing to discuss the drugs, and although he didn't quite recommend me to go and buy a copy of the BNF, he had no objection to my finding out about them. I think perhaps he realised, which some of the nurses didn't, that here was a bloody awkward customer and nothing was going to happen except by my agreeing to it. (p.150)

Working with clients

I'd like to paraphrase Piers Allott, who said something really valuable on this issue of working with clients in the previous chapter: recovery is essentially the job of the person who's had a mental breakdown or other mental health crisis: the role of the professional is to support that recovery process. Essentially, supporting a person's recovery means two things:

- holding out the hope that recovery is possible
- recognising the central place of self-management in recovery.

Supporting recovery may mean helping a person to identify what triggers their distress, as well as positive strategies for recovery that they have found work for them. It may mean helping them to develop an advance directive or statement about what they want to happen in a crisis. It may also mean a great number of other things, depending on the person and their needs. For example, it could mean pushing for in-depth therapy when this is required, or supporting a person in withdrawing from the psychiatric services, or from medication – if this is what they want. A growing number of resources on self-management are available, some of them online. One of the best established is the Wellness Recovery Action Plan (WRAP) programme, developed by Mary-Ellen Copeland, and mentioned by Piers Allott in the previous chapter. This and other resources are listed at the back of this book.

Challenging oppressive attitudes

Historically, people with a mental illness diagnosis were often not expected to recover. It's unfortunate that this view seems to have permeated the public consciousness, where it persists and contributes to the stigmatisation and oppression of those with mental health problems. It has also proved intransigent within psychiatric circles, as noted by several of my contributors, though there are now indications that things are beginning to shift. While it is inevitable that such views inhibit recovery from breakdown, the reverse will also be true. Telling people that recovery is possible as a matter of routine would be an enormously helpful and hope-inducing policy, which can be easily adopted on an individual basis.

Mental health professionals can also help a great deal by finding ways to challenge oppressive attitudes towards people with mental health problems in the wider world. This might mean meeting with local user groups to find out how best to help, as recommended by Phil Thomas in the previous chapter. It could also mean making small efforts on behalf of individuals, such as supporting a former client's application for employment. This is Jane:

> You try getting a job with a record like mine. Absolutely impossible... Psychiatrists tell you to lie. It makes me so angry that all they can offer their patients in terms of getting rid of stigma is to lie on a CV. (p.32)

Challenging oppression above all means confronting ignorance about mental health whenever it arises: in conversation with friends or colleagues, in the newspapers, or on the radio or television. Most important of all, this means checking our own attitudes and how we relate to other people in distress.

Grounds for optimism

The stories in this book – like all personal testimonies of severe mental health crises, are often deeply disturbing, but they are also illuminating. They show in graphic detail what it can mean to have a breakdown. They also show some hopeful outcomes, and information about what might help in a mental health crisis and what might not.

Overall, there are several grounds for optimism. From a personal perspective, the first is that mental breakdown can be a clearing house for positive change – as it was for me and for many others who have told their stories here. This is not to deny the suffering involved in a breakdown, but rather to reframe 'breakdown' as 'breakthrough'. Here's a word on this from Cheryl:

> Once I'd had the breakdown my attitude to myself changed. I seemed to have a clearer mind, and I started to see that I wasn't mad and that there was nothing wrong with me, that it was 10 years of pressure and no outlet... It was the counselling that really was the turning point for me, and one can only regret that I didn't have it earlier. (p.39)

Second, such experiences can make us a stronger person, more self-aware and more able to deal with our issues as they arise. Paradoxically, they can help us to come into our own, by spurring us to move in a more satisfactory direction work-wise or relationship-wise, rather than staying stuck – as so many do – in an unsatisfactory relationship or job. Maybe it's even true that people who have had these extreme experiences may look back on them as enriching. Third, they can dramatically broaden our understanding of human suffering in general, and increase our empathy towards others in distress. So there can be many positive spin-offs, and it can be helpful, as Graeme observes, to identify the benefits:

> I think I'm probably a lot more self-confident with meeting new people since I was ill than I was before... It does teach you a bit about human nature... [So] one can identify benefits and I think one has to because you'd get thoroughly fed up if you didn't. (p.154)

Further grounds for optimism are discernable from a broader perspective. In particular, there are many encouraging signs that things may be beginning to change significantly in the mental health services. The appointment of a recovery advisor on mental health to the Department of Health was one indicator; a growing number of mental health conferences and publications on the theme of recovery is another, though we need to be diligent that 'recovery' does not get co-opted into the medical model.

The positive signs of change are both a logical outcome of an increasing consumer-orientation of the health service generally, and a reflection of the impact of a growing mental health recovery movement worldwide. All of it means that recovery from mental illness is now a hot topic. The development of truly recovery-orientated services would be an immensely progressive step, if their adoption could be encouraged. It would be fascinating to see how much more rapidly people could begin to recover in this more hopeful environment. Such developments are now starting. They have not come out of the blue, but are the culmination of gradual developments in the services over recent years. These have included increasing user involvement in design and planning of the services, an increasing recognition that people can and do recover from mental health crises outside of the services, and an increased willingness on the part of mental health workers to listen to mental health service user/survivor stories, as reflected in the burgeoning of literature and training courses in the field. This book is one small contribution to this growing movement.

References

Allott, P. (2002) *Discovering Hope for recovery from a British Perspective.* Leeds: NIMHE.

Allott, P., Loganathan, L. and Fulford, K.W.M. (2002) 'Discovering hope for recovery: a review of a selection of recovery literature, implications for practice and systems change.' In S. Lurie, M. McCubbin and B. Dallaire (eds) 'International Innovations in Community Mental Health', Special Issue, *Canadian Journal of Community Mental Health, 21* (3).

Anthony, W. (1993) 'Recovery from mental illness: The guiding vision of the mental health system in the 1900s.' *Psychosocial Rehabilitation Journal (16) 4:* 11–23.

Bentall, R.P. (ed.) (1990) *Reconstructing Schizophrenia.* London: Routledge.

Bock, T. (1999) *Lichtjahre, Psychosen ohne Psychiatrie.* Bonn: Psychiatrie-Verlag.

Boyle, M. (1993) *Schizophrenia: A Scientific Delusion?* London: Routledge.

Department of Health (2001) *The Journey to Recovery.* London: Department of Health.

Faulkner, A. and Layzell, S. (2003) *Strategies for Living. The Research Report. A Report of User-Led Research into People's Strategies for Living with Mental Distress.* London: The Mental Health Foundation.

Freire, P. (1970) *Pedagogy of the Oppressed.* New York: Continuum.

Mosher, L. and Burti, L. (1994) *Community Mental Health: A Practical Guide.* New York: W.W. Norton.

Parker, T. (1996) *The Violence of Our Lives: Interviews with Life-Sentence Prisoners in America.* London: HarperCollins.

Read, J. and Faulkner, A. (2001) *Something Inside so Strong. Strategies for Surviving Mental Distress.* London: Mental Health Foundation.

Sainsbury Centre for Mental Health (1998) *Acute Problems. A Survey of the Quality of Care in Acute Psychiatric Wards.* London: Sainsbury Centre.

Thomas, P. (1995) 'Editorial. A letter from the consulting room: On the nature of professional barriers.' *Journal of Mental Health,* 5: 327–32.

UK ECT Review Group (2003) 'Efficacy and safety of electroconvulsive therapy in depressive disorders: a systematic review and meta-analysis.' *Lancet,* 361: 799–808.

Wallcraft, J. (2001) *Turning Towards Recovery. A Study of Personal Narratives of Mental Health Crisis and Breakdown.* PhD thesis.

Williamson, M. (1992) *A Return to Love.* London: HarperCollins.

Further reading

Bazire, S. (2004) *Drugs Used in the Treatment of Mental Health Disorders: Frequently Asked Questions (4th edition)*. Salisbury: Fivepin Ltd.

Breggin, M.D. and Cohen, D. (2000) *Your Drug May be your Problem: How to Stop Taking Psychiatric Medications*. Cambridge, MA: Da Capo Press.

Lynch, T. (2001) *Beyond Prozac: Healing Mental Distress*. Ross-on-Wye: PCCS Books.

Mental Health Foundation Strategies for Living Report:
www.mentalhealth.org.uk/page.cfm?pagecode=PBBRMHS4

Mary-Ellen Copeland: Mental health recovery and Wellness Recovery Action Plan

(WRAP) website: www.mentalhealthrecovery.com/

National Institute for Mental Health in England (NIMHE): www.nimhe.org.uk/

Newnes, C., Holmes, G. and Dunn, C. (eds) (1999) *This is Madness: A Critical Look at Psychiatry and the Future of Mental Health Services*. Ross-on-Wye: PCCS Books.

Newnes, C., Holmes, G. and Dunn, C. (eds) (2001) *This is Madness Too: Critical Perspectives on Mental Health Services*. Ross-on-Wye: PCCS Books.

Resources

Alcohol Concern

Alcohol Concern is the national agency on alcohol misuse, supplying information and details of local services. Based at: Waterbridge House, 32–36 Loman Street, London SE1 0EE. Tel. 0207 928 7377. Website: www.alcoholconcern.org.uk

Alcoholics Anonymous

Alcoholics Anonymous is a fellowship of men and women who share their experiences to stay sober and to help others recover from alcoholism. Contact via: P.O. Box 1, Stonebow House, Stonebow, York YO1 2NJ. Tel. 01904 644026 (office and helpline, Mon–Thurs 9.00–5.00, Friday 9.00–4.30). Website: www.alcoholics-anonymous.org.uk

British Association for Counselling and Psychotherapy

The British Association for Counselling and Psychotherapy provides information and advice on counselling and counsellors in the UK. Based at: 35–37 Albert Street, Rugby, Warwickshire CV21 2SG. Tel. 0870 443 5252. Website: www.bacp.co.uk

CRUSE Bereavement Care

CRUSE is a national voluntary organisation offering bereavement counselling and advice to all bereaved people. Branches in all areas. Contact via the local telephone directory or Tel. 0208 940 4818. Website: www.crusebereavementcare.org.uk

Depression Alliance

The Depression Alliance provides information, support and advice for those who suffer from clinical depression and their carers; also a network of self-help groups. Based at: 35 Westminster Bridge Road, London SE1 7JB. Tel. 0207 633 9929 (answerphone only). Website: www.depressionalliance.org

Eating Disorders Association

Information and help on all aspects of eating disorders, telephone support line and networking. Based at: 103 Prince of Wales Road, Norwich, NR1 1DW. Tel. 0870 770 3256. Fax 0160 366 4915. Helplines 01 603 621 414 (open 9.00 to 18.30 weekdays), Youthline 01 603 765 050 (open 16.00 to 18.30 weekdays). E-mail: info@edauk.com Website: www.edauk.com

Hearing Voices Network

Promoting understanding and tolerance for those who hear voices. Based at: 91 Oldham Street, Manchester, M4 1LW. Tel. 0161 834 5768. E-mail: hearingvoices@care4free.net Website: www.hearing-voices.org.uk

Manic Depression Fellowship (MDF)

The Manic Depression Fellowship is a national charity established by and for people whose lives are affected by manic depression. It provides a specialist advisory and information service, and has a network of self-help groups throughout the country. Based at: 8–10 High Street, Kingston-upon-Thames, Surrey KT1 1EY. Tel. 0208 974 6550. Website: www.mdf.org.uk

Mental Health Foundation

The Mental Health Foundation provides information and publications on a wide range of mental health issues and learning disabilities. Based at: 83 Victoria Street, London SW1H 0HW. Tel. 020 7802 0300. Scotland Office: 5th floor, Merchants House, 30 George Square, Glasgow G2 1EG. Tel. 0141 572 0125. Website: www.mentalhealth.org.uk

Mental Health Media

Works to reduce the discrimination and prejudice surrounding mental health issues and learning difficulties. Based at: 356 Holloway Road, London, N7 6PA. Tel. 0207 700 8171. Fax: 0207 686 0959. Email: info@mhmedia.com Website: www.mhmedia.com

Mind (The National Association for Mental Health)

Mind provides information and publications on mental health issues and services. Over 200 local Mind associations offer a range of day-care and other services. Contact via: Granta House, 15–19 Broadway, Stratford, London E14 4BQ. Tel. 0208 519 2122. Website: www.mind.org.uk

National Self Harm Network

Campaigns for the rights and understanding of people who self-harm. Contact: P.O. Box 16190, London NW1 3WW. Website: www.nshn.co.uk

Relate

Relate provides couples counselling for breakdown within relationships. Local branches throughout the UK. Based at: Herbert Gray College, Little Church Street, Rugby, Warwickshire CV21 3AP. Tel. 01788 573241. Website: www.relate.org.uk

Rethink, formerly the National Schizophrenia Fellowship (NSF)

Rethink provides information and services for people with a diagnosis of severe mental illness, especially schizophrenia, and their families and carers. The website also has lots of good information on recovery at www.rethink.org/recovery and links to the Rethink self-management project, email: selfmanagement@rethink.org. Rethink is based at: 28 Castle Street, Kingston-upon-thames, Surrey KT1 1EY. Tel. 0208 547 3937. Website: www.rethink.org

Samaritans

The Samaritans provide a confidential listening service for people who need to talk to someone. Listed in the local telephone directory, or telephone 08457 909090 or 08457 909192. E-mail: jo@samaritans.org. Website: www.samaritans.org

Scottish Recovery Network

Set up to promote and support recovery from long-term mental health problems, the Scottish Recovery Network aims to raise awareness about recovery, build an understanding of what helps recovery, and support examples of good practice. A key strand of their work is a narrative research project including up to 70 recovery stories. Website: www.scottishrecovery.net

Turning Point

Turning Point provides help and advice on problems with drink, drugs, mental health and learning disabilities. Based at: 101 Backchurch Lane, London E1 1LU. Tel. 0207 702 2300. Website: www.turning-point.co.uk

United Kingdom Advocacy Network (UKAN)

UKAN aims to promote advocacy and service-user empowerment, and to link mental health user groups nationally. Based at: 14–18 West Bar Green, Sheffield S1 2DA. Tel. 0114 272 8171. Fax. 0114 272 8171. E-mail: ukan@can-online.org.uk Website: www.u-kan.co.uk

Witness, formerly Prevention of Professional Abuse Network (POPAN)

Charity helping people who have been abused by healthcare or social care professionals. Based at: 1 Wyvil Court, Wyvil Road, London SW8 2TG. Tel. 0207 622 6334. Fax. 0207 622 9788. E-mail: info@popan.org.uk Website: www.popan.org.uk